MW00597502

RUNAWAY MOM

A Race to Regain My Sanity after Bipolar-Induced Postpartum Psychosis

Maggie Reese

Copyright © 2017 Margaret Reese. All rights reserved, including the right of reproduction in whole or in part in any form.

The author is donating a portion of the proceeds from this book to NAMI, the National Alliance on Mental Illness

Disclaimer: This book is intended to be informational, not a medical manual or medical advice. The author's comments are not intended to be authoritative, scientific, researched, nor a substitute for the advice and counsel or for any treatment or program that you may have been prescribed by your doctor. The advice and strategies contained herein may not be suitable for your situation. You should always refer any questions or concerns about your health to a trusted medical professional on whose advice you should rely. The information given here is designed to help you make informed decisions. This book is sold with the understanding that the author and publisher are not rendering medical, health, or other personal services. If you do not accept this understanding, please return the book for a full refund.

To guard privacy, names, biographical information, specific circumstances or dialogues, may have been changed. The mention of specific companies, organizations, or authorities does not imply endorsement or criticism by the publisher or author, not that they endorse this book.

While the publisher and the author have used their best efforts in preparing this book, they make no representations or warranties with respect to the accuracy or completeness of the contents of this book.

New Ideas Publishing and colophon are trademarks
of New Ideas Press.
For information regarding special discounts for bulk purchases,
please contact New Ideas Publishing Special Sales at
sales@NewIdeasPublishing.com.
NEW IDEAS PUBLISHING
BERKELEY, CALIFORNIA
Cover Photograph by Melissa E. Perkins
Manufactured in the United States of America

Published by New Ideas Publishing for Amazon
ISBN-13: 9781973483588

ABOUT THE AUTHOR

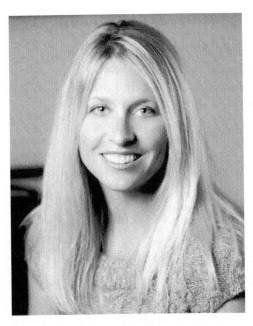

MAGGIE REESE

Maggie Reese's mission is to bring hope and inspiration to women facing mental illness or mental health challenges and their families and loved ones. In addition to sharing her personal stories in her books, Maggie speaks on how to live with mental illness, day-to-day coping skills, and the special issues relating to being a parent with mental illness. Maggie lives with her husband, Matt, and their daughter, Allison, in San Diego, California. Find Maggie on twitter @MaggieReeseAuthor.

DEDICATION

Dedicated to my Heavenly Father for the miracle of my sweet
AllieCakes

1

TABLE OF CONTENTS

Introduction

Part One: High Expectations Lead to Crash and Burn

Part Two: Limping Along on Three Cylinders

Introduction

There But for the Grace of God Go I...and any Mother

Post partum depression is an equal opportunity affliction.

It incapacitates celebrities like Brittany Spears. Linda Hamilton

and Hayden Panettiere. And it can hit the girl next door: ordinary,

loving, bright, beautiful moms like Maggie Reese.

Some new mothers survive postpartum depression or

psychosis. Others tragically do not. They may harm themselves and

sometimes their children.

Maggie did survive by the grace of God and through the

intervention and support of her family, caretakers and doctors.

Postpartum mood disorders are more common than you

may think. As many as 80 percent of new mothers experience mild depression within a year of giving birth. Up to 50 to 80 percent of all women experience some degree of emotional "letdown" following childbirth—the so-called "baby blues." Fortunately, the more extreme disorder, postpartum psychosis, is rare, affecting only about one in 1,000 new mothers.[1]

If you or someone you know has the baby blues it is still a serious condition and one where reaching out for help is vitally important. If the baby blues don't go away, they can lead to depression, which in turn can escalate to dangerous levels. In some situations, the depression can result in women experiencing psychosis and—in rare and tragic cases—can lead them to hurt themselves or their children.

If symptoms of baby blues persist for longer than two weeks, the mother should be evaluated to rule out the more serious mood disorder of postpartum depression, which is a mood

---

[1] https://womensmentalhealth.org/specialty-clinics/postpartum-psychiatric-disorders/?doing_wp_cron=1512518237.9291679859161376953125

disorder on the level of clinical depression. 12-16 percent of women experience postpartum depression, which results in feelings of despondency, inadequacy as a mother, difficulty in concentrating, memory problems and the loss of interest or ability to enjoy life.

Some of the symptoms of postpartum depression to watch out for include:

- Feeling "off" or just not like yourself
- Depressed or sad mood
- Tearfulness
- Loss of interest in usual activities
- Feelings of guilt
- Feelings of worthlessness or incompetence
- Fatigue
- Sleep disturbance
- Change in appetite
- Poor concentration
- Suicidal thoughts

If a pregnant women has any personal or family history of depression, Bipolar Mood Disorder, or Schizophrenia, it's important for her to tell this to her doctor. This history may *increase* her risk of developing postpartum depression or psychosis. By disclosing her history or other relevant factors during her pregnancy, she and her physician can work together towards an effective treatment plan should she develop a depressive or psychotic state of mind.

There is help for women with baby blues or the more serious postpartum depression. The place to start is by reaching out for help – to your family, your friends, your doctors. There are also many support groups and healthcare organizations that can help. We list many in the resource section at the end of this book.

Part One:
High Expectations Lead to Crash and Burn

Chapter 1

France

Mom and I were sitting on our balcony in Southern France in the town of La Roque Gageac on the Dordogne River. Our little house was made of stone. The back wall of each room was the rock cliff that vaulted over our heads. The first inhabitants had just piled rocks up against the soaring stone. And for over 400 years, people continued to live sheltered by the granite. The Dordogne. It was truly a magical place.

Pollen floated gently in the breeze casting a golden glow on the landscape. Mom painted non-stop while I looked with amazement across the verdant valley that swept down from the mountains up above to our little French home-away-from-home to the ancient town's winding streets and people going to and fro.

It was summer. High season. Crowded riverboats plied the river, music wafting up from the bands that serenaded the well-heeled tourists, lucky enough to escape the heat on the water. To my right there was a baronial estate, a maze of turrets and multi-levels of cobblestones. Off in the distance was an old castle, its grey façade shimmering in the late summer heat. Mom had chosen a special place to paint and for us to live - and I was glad to be here.

The only fly in the ointment was my stomach. The morning sickness was back. I was doing my best to try to control my queasiness, but I was spending much of my day around the toilet bowl - even now during my second trimester.

Besides the throwing up, I also felt that old fear creeping back. I had been off my medication for four months now. My head felt clear, but looming in the back of my mind was the question of whether or not my life was on the right path or not.

Back in San Diego I ran a modest day spa, but I was going to be letting it go. I knew I couldn't keep it going and concentrate on this new little being that was going to change everything in our lives. It was tough for me to come to terms with closing my business because I really liked my work. In the last few years, I had built up a steady clientele for facial treatments and massage. They filled my craving for constant social interaction and kept me grounded. It was scary to think of being home all day - with a baby - and it wouldn't be all about me anymore!

Yes, I was selfish. Part of me didn't want to life to change. Looking back now at the change I thought was coming and how I worried about it, I have to laugh at how unsuspecting I was about the impact I was soon to feel from the freight train of change that was barreling toward me, soon to run me over.

All of a sudden we were startled by a loud whooshing sound.

"Margaret - look up there. Oh, isn't it wonderful!"

About 100 feet above us, huge hot-air balloons appeared over the face of the cliff. Big red and yellow orbs of silk, thousands of little specks of pollen everywhere, French music drifting up from below.

"Mom, thanks for this trip," I said in a trance.

Just then I felt my baby move. It was so strange to think that I was actually going to be a mother. Since I was nineteen, doctors had been telling me that I should not have children. I had Bipolar Disorder, Type I, they would remind me. It would be a huge risk because you can't be on medication during your pregnancy.

Well, I didn't think pregnancy could be a big deal. I had been well for ten freaking years! I had followed doctors' directions

– so many doctors -- taken my medication, taken care of myself. What was all the hype about? Bipolar One - so what? I was managing it like a pro.

Again I felt the tiny kicking in my belly and smiled. My baby would be healthy. I would be healthy. What could go wrong! I wouldn't get sick, as so many doctors had warned me. I come out of this smelling like a rose. Think positive!

All the nay-sayers are nuts. I am going to be great and so is this baby inside me.

Everyone knows "denial" is a river in Egypt. Apparently it's in France too.

I looked up at the hot air balloons and waved to the people looking down at us as they floated by. It truly is magical where we are at this very minute. I know this will be my last big trip for a while. My mother keeps reminding me my life will come to a complete halt once this baby arrives. I'm going to enjoy myself and not listen to the worry.

My mother and I decide to pack a lunch and head off to see the famous carvings of the bulls. My mom says it is a "must see."

Road trips and morning sickness don't go well together. I am sick as all get out. All I can do is barf my brains out. I ask my mom to stop many times along the way to these special caves. I throw up, wash my mouth out, and then we continue.

I am very petite for being pregnant. I haven't gained much weight due to the constant nausea and I am 5'9," so I just have a little bump happening. My skin does have that characteristic glow and aside from my nausea, I feel surprisingly normal. I haven't had a normal feeling brain in over 10 years. It's a massive relief to not have my brain spinning 100 miles per hour every second of every hour of every day. Pregnancy is giving me an unexpected, but very nice break. I feel normal. Could I be cured? Will I never have to go back on medication? Did my pregnancy make my Bipolar go away? This is great. I can't wait to share the news with Matt and my doctors. Everyone with Bipolar I just has to get pregnant to get better. I will be written about in medical textbooks and journals. Maggie Reese and her baby cured Bipolar.

We get to Mom's very special caves and I now I feel like complete shit. I try my best not to complain because I know how important this is to Mom.

The Caves are called the Lascaux. These caves in Southern France are very famous. They feature cave paintings dating all the way back to the Paleolithic era. As I read the information given to us it tells us that these paintings are estimated to be 17,300 years old.

We enter into the caves and I immediately want to leave. I am feeling claustrophobic and a harsh anxiety come on. I don't like being in close quarters with all these French people. They are pushy and that sets me off.

Mom is in her glory so I try my best to stuff my crap away in my head. Slowly I start to appreciate how really incredible these works of art are. I start to calm myself with deep breathing and take in my mother's vibe and relax. We walk through the famous Rooms in the cave including the Hall of the Bulls, the Passageway, the Shaft, the Nave, the Apse, and the Chamber of Felines. The cave paintings are mind-blowing. I feel a touch of appreciation for what my mother is teaching me about art.

After touring the caves, we eat delicious French cheeses and yummy breads while mom paints. I rub my tummy.

The day is so hot I convince my mother to let me wade in the Dordogne River to cool off. I can't stop wondering what will happen when I get back to San Diego. Will my baby be okay? Will I be a good mother? I don't know the first thing about children so how will this all play out?

We spend the next day in the Doma. I am feeling especially sick and throw up with a bunch of French people watching. Just great! This is exactly what I need to start another day.

I decide to walk around the small hillside town while my mother sets up to paint. Her location is a perfect spot looking down on a valley full of vineyards, with the Dordogne River snaking through the center of the valley and picturesque chalets in the background. The scene is so vast and so beautiful I don't know where my mother will even begin to compose her painting for the day.

I start making my way through the village saying a cheerful "*bonjour*" to all the shopkeepers. Everyone is so busy here. I want to buy something for the baby. I find a cute little baby t-shirt to purchase and tuck it in my nap sack. I wonder about this little baby girl that is about to change my life forever.

Back at the vista my mother continues to paint an incredible picture of the valley below. She looks at me and smiles.

"Mags, why don't you paint a picture today?"

"Mom, I don't know how to paint."

"Just don't think about it", Mom encourages.

Mom takes my hand and puts a long paint brush in it and guides my hands with wide brush stokes across the clean, white canvas. Mountains begin to take form on the page, then the river below, the bridge in the distance, and the vineyards. Within an hour the picture has turned into the coolest thing I have ever created, with my mother's help of course.

"See, I told you so," mom says proudly.

We spend the next two weeks venturing around the Dordogne, our travels interrupted regularly so I can throw up. On our way home we decide to stay in Paris for a few days to take in the sights there.

I am really missing Matt by this time and can't wait to see him. I feel so fortunate to have Matt. He has been the love of my life since I was 19. Now at 31 here I am about to have his baby.

As we head to the Louvre to see Da Vinci's Mona Lisa and the famous Dying Slave by Michelangelo, all I can think about is how uncomfortable I am. It is so hot. I try not to complain but a few rude comments slide from my mouth. I hate this about myself. Here my mother is, giving me an incredible trip. I am in Paris for my last big trip before the baby comes and I complain about the dumb heat.

I wish I could relax and not think about myself, but it's not my nature. Perhaps my self-centeredness is a symptom of my disease. Most mothers innately put their children first. My mother has always done that. Once the baby is born, will we discover that I can put the baby first? Will my mother's traits be inside me after all? The uncertainty is a heavy worry weighing on me as the months of the pregnancy progress.

As we head into the Louvre I can see the excitement in my mother's eyes. Art is her world. She graduated college with a bachelor's degree in Fine Arts and English at Washington State in Pullman. We pass Monet, Matisse, and take in Pierre Bonnard. I know how important his work is to my mother so I stay quiet as she looks at each painting with awe.

The sketches by Vincent Van Gogh captivate me. I suspect that the reason I am drawn to Van Gogh's work is that I am aware of what we share. To me, it is a huge connection. We both have are have been burdened with Bipolar Disorder. It is the illness that will follow me to the ends of the earth no matter how much I pretend to be well or to follow the rules of society. It is always staring me in the face. I think about how often this ugly illness has won. It has killed so many. I don't want to end up dead like Van Gogh. I don't want to lose my mind ever again. Losing it once at 19 was bad enough. I have been through too much to ever get sick again. I have survived two mental institutions, looked into the face of death many times, and in ten years, have already taken more medication than a dozen people would take in their lifetimes combined.

As I look at a self-portrait of Vincent Van Gogh I can see the fear in his eyes. This gives me chills. I know that look too well. It is the look that says losing your mind is the most terrifying thing that can happen. He knows this. He knows what it is like to be locked up. He had been there, just like me. Looking through the bars and seeing the world go by. I shake off these bad thoughts that penetrate my soul and go around the next corner to find my mom admiring the Venus De Milo.

After the Louvre we decide to eat at a wonderful cafe right on the Seine. Our table overlooks the lights of the city and the swiftly running river below. In *bas relief* against the lilac twilight sky, Paris' ancient and modern buildings sit juxtaposed, the old world facing the new.

Our view is breathtaking. We eat to our hearts' content. For once this baby lets me not throw it all back up.

My mother takes a picture of me in front of the Eiffel Tower, Notre Dame Cathedral, the Arc de Triomphe, and we even hit a flea market where I decide to buy some lacy underwear as a gift for Matt. He will like these for sure.

Matt and I have always had great chemistry and no complaints in the sex department. We have sex just about every day even though I am as big as a house.

That evening my mom finds a delicious eatery where we have steak, mushrooms, and mashed potatoes. It is one of the best dinners I have ever had. On the plane ride home I am sicker then ever. I throw up all the way home. As we arrive in San Francisco my mother tells me, *"Well Margaret, this has been a trip of throwing up on Plains, Trains, Automobiles.... oh, and the River Boat!"*

~Reflections from Maggie's Mom~

Probably you are asking yourself "What on earth is this woman doing - taking a pregnant girl to France for Pete's sake"?

Well - this is why. As a little girl, Maggie "worked well" for food, expectations, and diversions - not necessarily in that order. She could be coaxed up that last ridge on a backpacking trip with the promise of M&Ms. The expectation of winning was the driving force behind her racing career - and she can still tell you every detail of every amazing meal she has ever eaten! So, the horse is out of the barn (so to speak). We have nine months to somehow get through without medication. What can I offer that is diversionary, raises high expectations, and has good stuff to eat? A trip is the perfect answer to all three - and since I had wanted to go to France in just forever - it seemed perfectly reasonable to me!

We would go in July - giving Maggie three months to "plan, organize, and have some wonderful expectations occupying her days". And she would be done with morning sickness, or so we thought. It's really hard to be happy when you are throwing up every other minute - but I assured her it would pass - and then we would leave on our trip.

She told me in May that the vomiting seemed to be passing - and every day she felt great - so I made the plans and we took off.

Somewhere over Greenland that part of the plan backfired! Probably she never had quit throwing up - but maybe she just started again… I will give her the benefit of the doubt I guess. I would have fibbed to go to Paris too!

I have to hand it to her - she was a trooper. She was sick on the train down to Brive. Once in the rental car, if I stopped alongside the road only once every ten miles it was a good day. I learned to be careful with the "food part" of the diversions - why buy expensive food when we were just going to see it again!

The caves of Lascaux were everything I had hoped. To see the first recorded site of man's attempt to draw not just what he saw - but to try to draw "power" or "beauty" or "fast" or just the "honor" of a thing was so marvelous that I just literally couldn't speak about it. (Maggie was awfully quiet too - and I am so glad that she began to understand why it was so important to me.)

It was hot - and the only way I could keep things together most days was to take her down to the river and plop her in it for hours. Fortunately, a river in France is a fine thing to paint. She pleaded for a trip with the other tourists on one of the big boats going up and down all day. They were expensive and I went from one company to the next, trying to find a reasonable one. We finally got on a likely looking boat - pushed off into the river and pushed right back in. Maggie up-chucked over the side and the boatman decided we were expendable.

Maggie thinks we were in France for 2 weeks - we were only there for 10 days - but hey - I had the diversion thing going just fine. In Paris, outside the Louvre and the Musee d'Orsay I gave her a talking to - somewhat along the lines of -*"I really need to do this"* - *"I have been wanting to come here since I was in college"* - *"if you have to throw up, you have to leave and I don't want to know about it, You will just have to wait for me outside no matter how scary that is"* …blah, blah, blah! In the end, I had a wonderful time - best all time ever - and Maggie did just fine.

So France worked! We used up three to four months. Maggie was doing fine off the meds - the extra hormones seemed to be working on her brain just fine. It was wonderful to see her eyes clear - the real her peering out again. In short, we had a wonderful time that will be in my memory forever.

Chapter 2

Nesting

After I returned home from my trip to France with Mom, instead of looking forward to my baby coming, I was full of dread and fear. I had a persistent, uneasy feeling that everything was not going to be okay, that I would be a failure as a mother. I kept on trying to talk myself through these strange feelings. I kept myself very busy getting the nursery ready, weeding my garden, and making arrangements at work to close up my little skincare and massage business.

For ten years my life had been darn awesome. I had lived at the beach for seven years, married Matt, opened my own business, got a beautiful yellow Labrador we named Jackson, and traveled all over. Matt and I had the perfect life together. Everything was about to come to a drastic change in about a month or so and that scared me to the core.

I really didn't know if I could do this mom thing. We had planned on not having children. Our plan was to travel our entire lives and work. Of course I always wanted to have a child growing up but after all the doctors told me I was high risk I had stuffed that dream away. Having a child when you were Bipolar 1 was very perilous.

I couldn't sit still in my tiny little house so I decided to mow the lawn. Something about cutting the grass always seemed to calm my brain. As I pushed the mower, I was sure I looked pretty silly to our neighbor Mark who was tending to his garden out front.

"Hey Maggie, take it easy", he said.

"Yeah, not to worry, Mark," I called out. *"I have at least a month left before I will be down for the count."*

I had my pink tank top on that no longer fit my very pregnant belly and jean shorts whose stretchable waistband was maxed out. I pulled the starter and the mower hummed to life. Back and forth I went making the lawn look great again. If only my life was this simple right now.

Less then a year ago I was turning 30. I had decided to have a fun birthday bash downtown. I saved up 500 bucks to pay for dinner for 15 of my friends at a Hawaiian restaurant called the Mr. Tiki's Mi Thia Lounge. It seemed like the fitting place for my party since Hawaii was one of my favorite places to vacation. My birthday went as planned with lots of awesome food, drinks, friends, dancing, and great sex with my husband at the end of the night. The only thing I didn't plan on was getting pregnant.

I was always very careful with birth control, taking my pills every day, and using condoms too. I had many conversations with my mother and doctors about how important this was. I didn't have the option so many others did, where getting pregnant was okay. To control my moods, I was on enormous amounts of Depakote - 2500 Milligrams to be exact. Who knew what this medication would do to a developing baby, and who knew what going off it would do to my sanity. No, getting pregnant was not an option for Matt and me.

Six weeks later, Matt and I were in South Lake Tahoe at his parents' vacation home on a ski trip when I began to feel strange. My menstrual cycle was always regular but I was a week late. My breasts started to hurt, and I was on an emotional roller coaster.

I told Matt I was very concerned I might be pregnant, but he felt I was worrying over nothing.

"Maggie calm down. How many times have you bought those silly tests over the years because you are so freaked out all the time?"

"Matt, I know my body and I think this time I really do feel that I am pregnant", I responded, too loudly.

"Mags, it's okay. I know you better then anybody. You never miss your birth control. So there is nothing to worry about. Now go get your snow gear on so we can get on the mountain."

I tried my best to believe him but my worry grew with every hour. I couldn't enjoy the snowboarding as usual because of the stress. I needed to go buy a test. I decided I would get one on the way to my parents in Jamestown.

We snowboarded Heavenly Ski Resort for the next three days. My body seemed to be more tired too. I was so relieved to leave the snow behind and head to the ranch. I had Matt stop at a liquor market on the way home where I found a pregnancy kit in the back aisle. I decided to buy two kits, which cost me way too much, but I needed some back up. I felt sure I was pregnant.

By the time we got to my parents' house, I marched right upstairs to the bathroom and peed on the small white stick. Sure enough, within a minute the telltale pink lines appeared.

I knew the test was right, but just to be doubly sure, I tore open the other box and took another test. It came out the same.

I couldn't believe it. This was *not* good. How could I have let this happen? I told my mom I wouldn't let this happen! I knew the risks.

Anybody else would be feeling pure joy at this very moment. Not me. I was in a state of pure panic and sadness. My life was at risk.

My heart was beating crazy-fast. Sweat started to bead all over my forehead and my hands began to tremble. I started scratching at a scab on my cheek in a feverish fit. Blood trickled down my face. My entire body felt out of sorts.

I felt as if my life was over.

"*Matt*," I yelled over the balcony. "*Can you please come upstairs really quick?*"

I felt a trickle of sweat run down my face. Or was it my tears? I knew Matt would freak out. He wanted children very badly, but at the same time, knew it was out of the question with me. We both had read all the information over the years about what a massive risk it was for me to get pregnant. I could hear him coming up the stairs and in about 30 seconds I would deliver the news that would change his life forever.

"*Mag, what is it?*" he asked.

I paused one last minute then said, "*Well, I was right. I am pregnant.*"

Matt dropped to his knees. He was in shock just as I thought he would be. He didn't say a word.

"*Well, aren't you going to say something,*" I said in a worried voice.

"*Mag, I can't believe it. Are you sure?*" he said shakily.

"*Of course I'm sure, you silly,*" I said. "*I took two tests. See, look at both of the boxes.*" I held out the torn boxes and the sticks.

Matt's head went to the side and his mouth was open with his hand on his head. He was pale and looked totally stressed. Instead of telling me it was going to be okay and hugging me he said, "*Maggie, are you going to be okay?*" He knew this could be the end of our happy life.

For most married couples this would be a joyous occasion and one they'd look forward to sharing with family, with hugs and cheers all around. But for us, our first thought was the fear of me losing my mind. It was almost too much to take in.

Instead of showing Matt my insane fear I said, "*Matt, I am totally going to be okay. It will be amazing. We are going to make great parents! Lets go tell my parents! They will be so happy for us.*"

"*Are you sure Mag? What about your Bipolar? How will this work? How can you take your medication?*"

He kept going on belting out questions. I just waved them off with simple answers and convinced him that I would be wonderful and no harm would come to our baby or me.

We headed downstairs, hand in hand, to tell my parents our big news. I was wearing my favorite tight, black shirt. I looked down at my belly seeing not a trace of the baby that was forming inside me. Maybe my mother would take the news okay. I guess there was only one way to find out.

My dad was putting some logs in the wood stove while my mom was making the gravy for her famous pot roast.

"Hey Mom and Dad, Matt and I have some news we want to

share with you!"

I tried to sound very confident in my delivery, but my voice

did crack when I said "*pregnant*".

My father tried to put on a good face like I did.

"Margaret, that is great, but what about your Bipolar,

Honey? This is so serious. You can't take your medication for the

next 8 months!"

My mother was not happy. Her voice was breaking as she

said: *"Pregnant! This is so scary for us all."* I knew what she meant

by this: that the very sanity I had held onto for the past ten years

was at stake. My family's lives could be tossed back into trouble

too. Yes, there was the fear staring us all in the face.

Mom was not taking this well at all. Her eyes narrowed into

that slant look she did when things looked impossible.

I kept telling her that I had been well for ten years and this was no big deal. This was going to be the best thing that ever happened to all of us.

Down deep I knew things were going to get very rough. I wasn't sure how hard, but I knew it was going to be a fight to have this child.

"Well Mags, you'd better call Carrie", my mother said. As I dialed Carrie's number I could hear my father tell my mother to calm down and that things would shake out alright.

If felt like it was taking forever for Carrie to answer her cell phone. Finally I could hear her voice on the other end. Carrie was my best friend. She had been with me through thick and thin since we were seven. She had survived my manic episode when I was nineteen and dispensed enough grace to last a lifetime. I was not prepared for her response either.

"Carrie," I said. *"I have some big new to tell you!"*

"*What's up Mag?*" she said.

"*Well, I wanted to tell you right after I told my parents: Matt and I are going to have a baby!*"

The silence on the other end of the phone line was deafening. "*Carrie are you there?*" Still more silence. "*Carrie!*"

"*Yes, I am here*", she said quietly.

"*I thought you would be excited, Carrie*", I said in a disappointed tone.

"*Mag, you know why I am not happy. You are not supposed to have a baby, remember? What is going to happen to your head?*"

"*Carrie, calm down. Sheesh! You and my mom are overreacting. I am totally going to be fine.*"

Carrie said she'd be as supportive as she could, but I could hear the reluctance in her voice and knew she was worried just like everyone else.

Next, we headed over to Matt's parents to share the news with them. They turned out to be overjoyed, a more normal response, but they were not thinking how terribly serious this was for me. Matt's parents were completely loving, but they hadn't been through all the doctor appointments and conferences my parents had gone to over the years, or heard the awful news about how risky it was for a woman with Bipolar 1 to have a child.

The list of negatives was so long for Bipolar mothers that I had put having children out of my mind. From getting pregnant with medication in your system, to the debate of whether or not to take meds during the pregnancy, to having a baby and not going crazy afterwards. All was fair game.

Even if I were to make it through the pregnancy okay and have the baby, my doctors had thought it would be likely that the stress of raising a child would be enough to send me back to the mental institution. I knew all this but chose to bury it deep and pretend that none of this mattered anymore, that I was above Bipolar.

Back in San Diego I started telling all my friends, co-workers, and just about anybody I met that I was going to be a mom. I started to get excited about the idea instead of worried. I found a good female doctor I really liked too. She said I was 6 weeks along and everything looked great.

At about 9 weeks, I woke up with enormous pains in my stomach. Matt had already left for work as I limped to the bathroom. What was happening to me? I peed and wiped and was horrified to find blood all over the toilet paper.

No! This couldn't be happening. Not a miscarriage! I wanted this baby.

Over time I felt more cramping and more blood came out. I looked down at the toilet sadly, sing only tissue coming out.

I started to cry as I dialed Matt's cell phone. Matt came right home when I told him the news. He just held me while I sobbed. I then called my mother and felt dead. She was so positive and reassuring. She told me that if I wanted another baby that she was sure I could do it.

"Maggie, think of it as a new chance to get pregnant with no medication in your system and to get all the best help possible."

Maybe Mom was right. For the next week I didn't want to eat or do anything. I wasn't motivated to take care of my skin care shop and had no energy to massage anyone. I think my mom began to worry because the next thing I knew she flew down to be with me. She took me to eat at all my favorite restaurants and bought me a couple of cute outfits to cheer me up.

Matt was also trying to process this unexpected loss. Within the few days of Mom's visit I had made up my mind that I wanted to have a child more then ever. I would let this miscarriage go and look forward to getting pregnant once again. Only this time it would not be a mistake but would be on purpose!

My doctor thought it would be best to wait 2-3 months before we started trying. Matt and I skipped her advice completely and started trying right away. Within a month I was pregnant. This time I waited until my second trimester to tell everyone.

Matt was crazy in love with me and this baby. Our love for each other seemed more intense then ever before. We ended up having sex every day of my pregnancy. No joke!

We were given October 20th for the due date. Everyone was overjoyed and everything seemed to be right with the world. Maybe we were all worried but didn't want to show it to one another. Our happiness outweighed our fear of the unknown.

So now here I was in late September cutting grass to get ready for this baby. We had decided on a name for our baby girl. Her name would be Allison Isabelle Reese. Matt came up with it from the newspaper. Allison Hays was an actress in the 1950's in Hollywood. There was an article about her in our local paper that Matt happened to read. He loved the name and wanted to add Isabelle so her initials would be A.I.R. I loved the name too. How cool to have those initials, right! Like the Nike Airs I used to run in.

Allison Isabelle would be arriving soon enough. I rolled the lawn mower back in the garage and headed back into the nursery to see what else I could do. I looked at the crib with curiosity. What would take place in the months to come? Would I come out of this all right like I hoped? Would my little Allison be all right? I didn't even know how to change a diaper. Who was I kidding? I was scared to death. No wonder I was filled with so much dread in France. My life was about ready to shift whether I liked it or not. I'd better get everything ready to go. I started opening boxes of diapers and putting them under the changing table. I guess it was time to make a nest.

Reflections from Maggie's Mom

I thought there was one huge problem that no one was talking about - and since I couldn't figure out any good way to bring it up - I just let it go. Genetics!

When Maggie was diagnosed as Bipolar, the first Doctor had asked me if we had any mentally ill people in our families. As I recounted in Maggie's first book, *Runaway Mind*, to my horror, it was me that passed on that particular gene. In my family, my mother's brother, Uncle Jim, was Bipolar. A brilliant man who somehow managed to raise a good family, he was a chemist with a large company who valued him - and were supportive when he would have his "bad times". The only other member of our large family tree that seemed to be a possibility was my mother's father's older brother, Uncle George. He died walking on a train track - and the suspicion was that it was not accidental.

If there were more relatives with Bipolar in preceding generations, they are lost in our knowledge. While I have a pretty well filled out family tree, it doesn't say whether or not any of them had mental problems. That's the kind of information that doesn't get passed on.

When I found out about "my complicity" in Maggie's illness, I could not help but think about another possibility. When I was having babies, I did not have an easy time of it. My first pregnancy ended in a miscarriage.

We waited 3 months and tried again. Unlike the first time, this time I sick every morning for 3 months and Amy Anne was born 9 months later.

When we decided to increase our family, I had three more pregnancies in a row - all three times ended at about 10 weeks with a miscarriage. I never was sick. The doctors just said try again. I do remember a well-meaning neighbor telling me that sometimes there was something wrong with those babies, and someone else said miscarriages were God's way of "taking care of things".

Long story short, - pretty soon I was pregnant again - and throwing up mightily -every morning and so glad for it! Margaret Ruth was the happy result and then two years later Thomas Josiah showed up - me losing my lunch at every opportunity!

So - were my "other" babies not good ones? Should I have not tried so hard? Did my body just "weed out" problem babies? Was God trying to tell me something and, because I didn't listen, my Maggie was born with this terrible condition?

I dealt with these questions in my own way - and went on with my life. But in my case I had the "Well - we didn't know" defense going for me. Now we did know - and that meant a whole new level of obligation.

Were these two kids going to be able to handle the same question? Matt has some mental illness issues in his own family tree - and according to everything I have read, that is not a good thing either. The more "instances" on both sides, the more chances that children will have the condition. I had to assume that they both knew the risks.

Of course, some doctors don't agree at all - they say genetics has only a small part in Bipolar.... but for me, and for my family, I think it does.

When Maggie lost the first baby, I admit it, I was relieved. Then I realized how terribly down she was – scared-me-out-of-my-mind low - so I went down to stay with Maggie for a week. I went through all my "bag of tricks" - the food, the new clothes, and tried to give her advice to go to her doctors, both the physical and the psychiatric, and listen to what they told her. In short, I bucked her up and got her going again - so I wasn't too surprised when they were in business in the baby department again.

One last note - I might have hated all the vomiting in France, but secretly I was so glad - to me it meant that THIS baby was going to make it into the world!

Chapter 3

Times Up!

October 2006 ~ Three weeks before our baby girl was to be born I got quite a surprise in the middle of the night.

"*Matt get up,*" I shouted! "*Allison is coming. She is ready to get out!*"

Matt just rolled on his side and said, "*Babe, go back to sleep, she is not due for three more weeks!*"

"*Matthew, get up now, and I mean now. I am leaking all over myself and it is not pee!*"

"Call my doctor. Get up!!" I shouted. That finally got his attention. He was throwing things in a suitcase. Our dog Jackson started barking, and I just got a big smile on my face!

I was ready for this baby girl even if she was a little early. Don't get me wrong though. I did love being pregnant. It made me feel fantastic. I had not felt that normal since I was 18! Living with Bipolar Disorder had been rough all these years and for some wonderful reason I was able to live life like a normal person during my pregnancy. Maybe it was all those hormones that change your body for better or worse. For me they worked like a charm. I would joke with friends I just needed to stay pregnant then I wouldn't have Bipolar anymore!

I did have my concerns though and my parents very worried from the get-go. Mom and I had gone to conventions and heard doctors say that it would be high risk to have a child and a challenge to stay sane. But for some reason I had talked myself into believing that I was past this whole mental illness thing and I could do what anyone else could.

Matt pretty much went along with what I thought because he wanted a baby so much too. So off we went to the hospital in La Jolla in the middle of the night. Little did I know when I came back to our cute tiny bungalow life would be different in every way. Nothing would ever be the same.

As we went up the hospital elevator I continued to leak amniotic fluid all over the place, but I didn't care. I was too excited about having this baby. Matt was squeezing my hand so hard I thought it just might fall off! The nurse took us to the delivery room and they hooked me up to all kinds of machines.

Matt started the phone calls and I settled into being content with the pain. I am good with pain so the contractions were not too much for me to handle. The doctor said I was only 1 cm dilated so she wanted to get things moving with the Pitocin. I just remember

nodding and saying yes to whatever they wanted to do.

Unfortunately it was not an easy delivery. At 18 hours I was still

only 1 cm and my only option was an emergency C-section. I was a

little scared but what else could I do? I remember my sister was

there by then and my mom had just driven from a trip she was on

in Las Vegas. I was done with all the pain by that time so it sounded

like a fine thing to do.... GET THIS BABY OUT!

Matt and my mom got to be in the delivery room with me.

The C-section went smoothly although I was pretty out of it. I

guess I made the doctors laugh with some of my wild tales. Matt

almost fainted but hung in there with a nurse's help, sitting for just

a minute. Matt fell in love with Allie immediately and was able to

cut her cord. I got to see our Allison Isabelle Reese just a minute,

and then she was taken for all the follow up care. Mom was there

with tears and hugs. My sis looked through the window with a smile. I felt loved and had given my heart to this little baby that I had just met for the first time.

The early days after Allie's birth were peaceful and magical. After recovery I was put in my own room with an incredible view of the hot air balloons going by. Funny@ Here again, seeing the balloons and being in such an amazing place in my life!

Just then a cheerful, pretty nurse walked in. *"Hi Maggie, I'm Danielle. I will be your nurse for the next few days and I am going to get you breastfeeding right now!"*

Wow, I thought to myself. This is wild. I don't know how to do that! Well, let me tell you, Danielle picked up my little peanut, put her to my breast, Allie snuggled right onto my nipple and latched on right away, and there you go - I was feeding her! The baby's instincts met my body's innate physical responses perfectly and effortlessly. Would this be how motherhood would feel, and how it would go?

There was something about Danielle that just made me had a connection with her right away. Beyond a nurse relationship. I just had this feeling we would be friends beyond the hospital.

Family came and went to meet little Miss Allison and Matt was in happy father heaven.

I felt great but maybe a little off. I remember thinking it must be just because I was so tired.

> FIRST MISTAKE: I had planned to get back on my Depakote after I breastfed for a while.

> SECOND MISTAKE: I wasn't taking any sleeping medicine at night because of nursing the baby.

> THIRD MISTAKE. There were no breaks for me ever.

By about the fourth day in the hospital I started to get manic. I didn't realize that I was acting strange, but my mother knew right away. She said she saw my eyes and knew there was going to be trouble - Big Trouble.

Everyone else kept saying that I was just so excited about the new baby but Mom knew that look, that sound in my voice. I remember seeing the worry in her face and thinking, why is she staring at me that way when I have this amazing little baby and I am all right.

My nurse Danielle knew of my past breakdown when I was first diagnosed with severe Bipolar disorder 1 because my mother and I had told her the story of my first episode at 19. As a runner, I had gone off to the University of Idaho on a full-ride athletic scholarship and within months my world had crashed into utter destruction.

I told Danielle how I had written a book called *Runaway Mind* and that one day I wanted to publish it. Danielle was impressed by my story and said she was so moved that she just wanted to be there for me in every way she could. Before I left the hospital she too was concerned with the way I was acting. She gave me her number and said I could call anytime.

One other person who was pretty worried was my sister. She could see that wound-up look I had and the tension in my body.

I had gone into the hospital on a Sunday night and was now being wheeled out to the car on Friday afternoon. Having a C-Section I needed more time to recover.

As Matt pushed me down to the car waiting at the circular drive I remember feeling high as a kite, like I was some famous person and that everyone was looking at me because I had this beautiful baby. These are manic delusions to a "T."

Matt put our little peanut in the back of the Jeep in her cute little purple baby carrier. I sat beside her all excited, but thinking only of myself. Not really thinking that here I was this new mom and how much I loved this baby. This is hard to admit to and say, but it was true.

Matt and the rest of the family were all caught up in the excitement of Allison. There was so much going on that the fact that I was spiraling away was slipping between the cracks.

Chapter 4

Ride Home

We hit afternoon traffic going towards downtown San Diego. We were moving along at snail's pace. I couldn't stop laughing at everything Matt said. I didn't really think too much about cute little Allie sitting beside me. I'm sad to think that now, but back then my mind was going mad.

By the time we got home I was worn out beyond what seemed imaginable. Our yellow lab, Jackson, gave Allie a little lick to and then we were greeted by family who filled up every available space in our small, green, 1937 craftsman home. By small I am not kidding you...it was 732 square feet. It was an amazing little home though, with so much charm, and we still miss it! Matt's parents and my mom had set up a nice dinner for us. I was overwhelmed with how nice the house looked. The moms had done so much while we were away for the week.

For some reason I felt the need to check my e-mail. I went into my little office and my brain just started making up stuff like crazy. It was a delusion, but I thought for sure that Matt's mom Donna had been reading all my e-mails. I shut down. I told Matt what I thought and whispered in a strange way that I would keep it together.

I went out to our little kitchen and pretended I was fine. Inside my mind was full of rage. I wanted to go tell Matt's mom to fuck herself and hit her. I tried with all the strength I had to keep from jumping across the table and choking her. When Matt's parents left I tried my best to stay calm. Mind you, this was all made up in my head. The sad thing is it seamed so real that I believed everything that I thought.

I tried breast-feeding the best I could. When my milk came in, it shocked me. Lets face it...things were changing in my body, mind, and soul. By the middle of the night I still was not sleeping. I got up to breast feed many times during that first night home and tried to calm Allie. My mom was sleeping on the couch and helped me through the night. I don't think either of us got any sleep.

Chapter 5

Mind Gone

The next day Matt went out to golf with his father, uncle, and cousin to celebrate in Coronado. By midday I had lost my mind entirely. *"Mom, Matt has died. I am finished without him,"* I cried.

"Maggie, Honey, what are you talking about?" said my mom, looking worried. *"He is golfing, he is fine."*

"No, Mom. I know he is dead. You don't know what I see."

I went on like this for what seemed liked eternity. Mom called Matt and reported the horrible news. *"Matt, get home right now! Maggie is very sick and we need to get her help right away."*

Mom called my psychiatrist but it was the weekend. There was only an answering machine. I was getting worse by the second, descending into a complete psychotic break.

I can't tell you how scary it is to think things are really happening but they are not. It makes my first episode back in 1996 look like a cake-walk. I thought there was an ambulance on its way to pick up Matt's dead body. I heard the sirens blaring in the distance as my mom kept trying to shake me out of my shocking state. I didn't hear a thing she said though and only looked down seeing Matt's motionless body before me. I had no awareness of the fact that I had a baby girl in the next room sleeping peacefully and that things really were all right. To me life was over. I had just lost the love of my life, my everything.

Matt came into my life at the young age of 14. He was the guy I had a crush on in junior high school. Later he would go off to boarding school and I would go to public high school. We would reconnect after my freshman semester at University of Idaho. I saw him at the movies with his dad and brother and was instantly attracted to him once again. I was with my high school boyfriend at the time so all I could do is wish that Matt was my boyfriend.

I would not see Matt again until we met up on a water-ski day trip later in the summer of 1996. Between the Christmas break sighting of Matt and the summer water-ski meet-up I had dropped out of University of Idaho twice and even tried to go to Cal Poly San Luis Obispo. I had been diagnosed first with depression and then later manic depression when I was hospitalized at the local mental hospital.

Then came the water-ski day. I was invited to go by Matt's brother and his friends. I was surprised that my mother let me go with Matt's brother, Todd, on the water-ski outing. At the time I was in the midst of my manic episode and had been out of the mental hospital for a few days in my hometown of Sonora.

My parents were in a massive panic. They couldn't keep up with my crazy ideas and never-ending energy, or with my being very rude and hurtful. They had already hired one of my old friends, Josh, from high school, to help babysit me, but he quit after three short days. Who could blame him? I was a nightmare in every way imaginable.

Matt wasn't at the outing nor was I looking for him or thinking about him. I was just glad to be with some old friends from my past at the local Adventist school I had attended in junior high.

That day Todd split his toe open very badly on some sharp rocks as we were jumping into the lake. I was instantly interested in all the blood that gushed from his toe as one of the parents wrapped it in bandages. It needed immediate attention at the ER and I wanted to be there to see what would take place.

All the commotion stimulated my already altered manic brain and I rode with Todd to the hospital. Somehow I was able to talk my way into staying with Todd as he was stitched up. I had no ride home nor did I want to go home so I asked if I could ride with Todd to his house and have my parents pick me up there.

I will never forget that day I walked into Todd's house. There was Matt lying on the couch watching sports. I knew I had to be with him. There was this crazy part of me that just had to be near him and I would do whatever it took to do just that.

I was able to get my parents to hire Matt to be my new babysitter or what I would later tell everyone else my bodyguard during my manic adventures. He kept me safe through my highs-

and lows until I would be forced to go to Stanford Psych Ward. On

my return from my 22 day stay at Stanford I would end up dating

Matt for six years and later marrying him in 2002.

I looked up and saw the fire trucks outside and the

paramedics rushing up to my home and pushed by my mother to

Matt's body. They put him on a stretcher and somehow got him

breathing, which was impossible because he had been dead at least

five minutes.

"*Mom,*" I screamed. "*I have to follow them.*"

"*Mags,*" she pleaded with me. "*There is nobody there. Trust

me honey everything is all right. Nobody is dead. You are with me

and Allison your baby girl.*"

I heard none of it. I just kept on going into this deep, dark

psychosis that I now was trapped in and only saw what my brain was making up. I heard the ambulance pulling away with Matt and the sirens fade.

In the meantime, Matt pulled up and ran up the steps into our tiny home. *"Maggie, look at me I am alright,"* he screamed.

I just stood there in a daze thinking he was not really there but some vision I was making up. I was so scared and confused. My body was trembling out of control and I couldn't figure out how to calm myself.

"Mags, honey, listen to me, we are all fine...look at our baby girl," Matt whispered.

There was no response from me. I was in another time another place. A world that I was completely trapped in. There was a small part of me that was trying to claw my way out of my madness but I was in it too deep.

"Matt, we need to get Maggie to the hospital. We have to get her medication and she might have to be hospitalized," my mother

said. With more phone call to my psychiatrist and just the answering machine picking up, Matt decided to call my OBGYN. Mom and Matt were able to reach Dr. Marshall and I decided that is the only way I would listen to anyone....if I talked with her.

"Dr. Marshall, are you listening? Do you hear what I am saying? I know things and see things that others can't but you can't tell. I can only discuss things through the papers." I rambled on like this for a few minutes and somehow Dr. Marshall was able to listen, stay patient, and then was able to talk me into going to the hospital for help. Matt got home and I hugged him but didn't really think he was living. I thought he was just a vision before me. I was scared out of my mind and could only think of going to the hospital to see if he was still living.

"Maggie, listen to me! I am all right. I am right here baby," Matt pleaded. Again I didn't believe what I was hearing.

"*Mags,* " Mom said. "*We have to get you dressed so Matt can take you to the hospital.*"

"*Hospital,*" I whispered. "*Is Matt going to be there?*"

"*He is going to take you honey. You are going to go get checked out. You will get through this.*"

I was so confused. Through this? What was my mom talking about? That Matt was dead or alive at the hospital. or is she saying that I am not all right. What was happening? Nothing made sense. I went in my room and started taking off my clothes.

"*Mags, sweets,*" mom said. "*You need clothes on to go to the hospital.*"

"*No Mom. If I take them all off Matt will live.*"

"*Maggie,*" Mom cried "*Please put on your clothes. You are going to be okay. We just need to get you help.*" So I started putting back on my clothes then instantly started stripping them all off.

My mind was so far gone by this point there was no reasoning with me and I couldn't figure out why I should have clothes on. My head killed, my body ached, and especially my stomach. I then felt where the pain was coming from. I had stitches going through my skin right above my vagina. What was that doing there? For a split second I thought well maybe that is where they cut me open to get my baby out. But just as the thought would flash through it would just as fast vanish. It was a disaster.

During all this, Mom or Matt was taking care of little baby Allie because I sure wasn't. At this point I think I had completely forgotten that I had a newborn.

I then tried to run out the door completely naked. I got to the front gate with my mother yelling after me. Thankfully I couldn't figure out how to open our small front gate and my mother tackled me and pleaded with me to come back inside. Unfortunately our neighbors saw all of this but they realized something was very wrong with me and helped my mother and Matt.

After 10 minutes of clothes coming off and on, Mom finally got me to leave my clothes on. Matt put me in the Jeep. On the way to La Jolla I kept muttering things that made no sense and I am sure Matt was probably in shock. Here he had just had this beautiful baby enter his life and within less then a week his wife was checking out of life completely.

Matt tells me now he had a sinking feeling it would be a long time before I would come back to the land of the living. My eyes were gone. Gone in a way that he said he would look at me and there was nothing there.

I didn't acknowledge him. I remember driving up the 5 south to the hospital and wanting to leap from the Jeep. I thought I could stop the car and go find Matt somewhere.

Chapter 6

Your Wife is on Drugs

The next thing I knew we were in the waiting room of the ER. I saw a drinking fountain and immediately went over to it and started drinking water. I couldn't stop. I thought if I did, Matt would die. I felt everyone watching me as I tried really hard to stay connected to the fountain. As I looked up at the room full of people I found they were looking at me with puzzled faces.

Matt called my name just then, *"Mags, please come to me. You don't have to keep drinking that much water."*

There was that tone again. A tone of worry and confusion.

Why was my world coming undone so quickly? Why was I here in

this place? Why did Matt look so sad?

With the help of a nurse I finally let go of the drinking

fountain and was guided into a room. My eyes were wide with

excitement and I couldn't stop moving. The nurse asked if I had

taken any drugs of any kind. I was insulted by this question,

especially since I had never had an illegal drug in my entire life.

"*NO, I haven't!*" I shouted back at her. "*I just had a baby a

few days ago, I have Bipolar 1, there is something wrong with me,*" I

stammered. The nurse just nodded like a bobble head character

and left the room.

"*Matt, tell me what is going on? What is wrong?*"

Matt gave me a huge hug and said, "*Mags, it's okay we are

going to get some medication and help and get you back. Just tell

them exactly how you are feeling and we can get the help you need.*"

Just then the doctor came in. *"Hi Margaret,"* I am Doctor

M. *"Tell me what is going on."*

I felt my face getting hot. I felt the anger rising from my

belly. I knew I needed to stay calm but I could not control myself.

"I JUST HAD A BABY AND I HAVE BIPOLAR," I shouted. *"I know*

exactly what is wrong with me. Just give me some medication so I

can go home and get well."

The doctor said a few things to Matt and then the nurse that

I couldn't make out. This angered me more.

"I am right here. If you want to talk about me. SPEAK up!"

Matt tried his best to calm me as I became more and more

agitated. I couldn't calm down though.

Time must have passed. Things happened, but I couldn't

make out what was happening. All of a sudden, Matt's mom and

dad were in the room speaking with Matt and the doctor. Were they really there? I couldn't quite figure out if they were there or not. Was my mind playing tricks on me? Things were very fuzzy.

Then I heard the doctor telling Matt I had tested a positive for drugs.

"*I AM NOT ON FREAKING DRUGS!*" I shouted at the top of my lungs.

Matt said, "*Mags, I know Honey. Doctor, you don't understand how seriously my wife has Bipolar. She has never done drugs. She never has touched any.*"

The doctor just said simply, "*I am sorry Mr. Reese but you need to take her to a drug rehab center where she can get the proper treatment.*"

Matt's dad must have been there because I could barely make out his voice talking with the doctor. I was livid. But then I spaced out and checked out completely. It was so odd because I knew there was something really wrong but I couldn't get out of the state I was in. My brain was like a light switch. One minute I could

understand what happening then the next moment it was back off

again.

Chapter 7

Chevy's

The next thing I knew we were in Mission Valley at Chevy's

Restaurant. I was trying to order something but I was confused. I

realized we had a baby with us. I thought it was mine but I couldn't

really tell. Matt was bending over the little being, playing with it.

What was going on? I felt really out of it.

I ate some chips and salsa and fought to get my bearings. I

needed more ice tea. *"Where is the fucking waitress?"*

I tried to sit still. I couldn't though. I wanted to run, but my

stomach hurt. I thought, *I am a mom. I think I had a C-section. I* slipped my hand around my lower area of my body. I felt the stitches.

Yes, that is it. I just had a baby a few days ago! That is my baby, Allison Isabelle Reese! I reached out to her in the little baby carrier. I felt like everyone's eyes were on me. So I grabbed back my hand with a start and folded my hands beneath the table. I didn't know how to be a mom and I was really ill. I felt myself going dizzy again and fazed out through the rest of the dinner or lunch or whatever meal it was, whatever time it was.

Chapter 8

The Bible ~ Really?

Back in my home my mother was waiting at the door. Her eyes had that odd slant to them again. I hadn't seen that expression for years. It was that one that said I was very sick and she was extremely worried.

I hated those eyes looking at me like that. I wanted to tear those fucking slant eyes out. I hated them. I hated that I felt like this. I was losing control of my thoughts again. How do I function? I was instantly enraged and wanted to tear my hair out. I started counting. Sometimes, at about fifty, my thoughts would calm down.

I needed to lie down for a few minutes to catch a small break from my thoughts. They seemed to be racing non-stop. John, Matt's cousin, was at the house working on the kitchen sink. I didn't want to talk with John or my mom so I quickly ran into the back bedroom and threw myself on the bed. I just needed my brain to slow for a few seconds so I could get back to my baby and Matt. I knew I was disconnected from life but couldn't figure out how to get back. I wondered if John thought there was something off. I needed to rest. I was angry, aggravated, and felt out of control. I needed to call Carrie. She would know what to do. She always does.

"*Hello Maggie,*" Carrie said.

"*Carrie, I am freaking out I can't handle my brain. Everything is so distorted. Tell me what to do,*" I said anxiously.

"*Mag, I know you don't care about the Bible, but I am going to give it to you anyways. Just listen really quick, okay Mag,*" she told me.

"Oh, the damn fucking Bible. What the hell is God going to do for a madwoman? I will tell you what -- Nothing. Fucking nothing, that is what." My jaws were clamped together and my head was pulsing.

I was angry with God. Why did he do this to me? Seriously, what did I do that is so wrong in my life to be this fucking ill? Everyone else gets to have a baby and enjoy it, but me.... every other second I forget I have one.

My veins were pumping adrenaline like crazy. I could hardly focus until Carrie recited the verse. It was from Philippians.

"Mag, just listen to me", she told me calmly.

"Do not be anxious about anything. But in everything by prayer and petition, with thanksgiving, present your requests to God. And the peace of God, which transcends all understanding, will guard your hearts and your minds in Christ Jesus."

My brain started to check out, but as Carried started to recite the verse, I snapped to attention. *"Thanks Carrie. That does help. I don't know why, but it helps,"* I told her.

I hung up with phone and feel at peace for a few good minutes. Maybe God was there. I didn't know. I couldn't decide. I wanted to scream to Him right now and yell, *"GOD, IF YOU ARE REAL THEN YOU NEED TO HEAL ME NOW!"*

The next thing I knew I heard my mom and Donna in a heated discussion about the computer. What were they so mad about? I plugged my ears and jumped under the covers because I couldn't take on any more stuff. I breathed long breaths. I thought Matt, Allie, and his dad must have been gone because all I heard were the moms getting all wound up, which made me cringe. I couldn't take all the noise. My hearing was all messed up. All my senses were heightened beyond what I could possibly take. I could hear sounds outside that I normally couldn't hear or shouldn't hear. Everything was just a bit too clear and loud. It caused my

head so much pain. I got under the covers and rocked myself back

and forth saying "*Jesus*" until I passed out.

Chapter 9

Shower Terrors

When I woke up it was dark. I needed to go to the

bathroom. I walked quickly to the restroom, went pee, and then

used an entire roll of toilet paper. My brain was going so fast I

couldn't remember if I wiped or not.

While on the toilet I looked down at the black and white

checkered floors. They needed to be cleaned. I flushed the toilet

and started scrubbing the floor with a hand towel. As I started

cleaning the floors the toilet then overflowed with all the toilet

paper I had just stuffed in it. I threw the towel down and walked

out. I saw my mom standing there but I pushed past her back to the bedroom. I turned around and asked if Matt was dead. She just looked at me with those eyes and said, "Margaret, Matt is fine. He is in the kitchen with Allie your baby Honey."

"*Oh right,*" I muttered, and then lay down on the bed again.

Oh those eyes. How awful they were.

Am I really that sick? I need to just be okay. Maybe if I lie here and take a little Klonopin to calm down I might chill out a little. I hate feeling like this. I am so irritated and mixed up at the same time. It makes me so upset to feel so stretched, so intense inside. I can't relax. Maybe I can rest if I breathe deep and close my eyes.

The next thing I knew it was the next day and Matt's cousin, John, was there doing plumbing on the toilet. I stopped it up pretty well. I could hear John and Mom talking away about me in the kitchen.

"*MOM,*" I yelled. "*I can hear everything you guys are saying. Please just go outside.*" They stopped and went out on the back deck with Allie of course. There was no way I could be left alone with baby Allie. Almost every other minute, I didn't even know if I had a baby.

My hair felt dirty and gross. In fact, I felt dirty. When was the last time I took a shower? I didn't know? Had it been a week? My skin was itchy. I started looking at my body in the mirror and was horrified by the way I looked. What I saw were sunken eyes, frazzled, oily hair, a bloated face, and the rest of my body was oddly distorted.

I guess any new mother might feel this way, but to me, I couldn't remember second to second that I had a child and that is why my body looked this way. It panicked me to no end that I had stitches just above my vagina. Somebody had cut me open. Why did they do this? Sometimes for a moment I would remember why and then the reality would be gone again and I would be left with the horror of the way I looked. My face had even broken out with pimples and my hairline looked as if I had pulled out my hair though really it was just that some of my hair fell out as sometimes happens after you have a baby.

I had to get in the shower. I felt like I was really dirty and my breasts hurt really badly. I immediately turned on the shower. Then my brain flipped another switch. I thought that something in the shower was going to kill me.

"MOM," I shouted! "*I can't get in the shower. The water is trying to get me. Please help me,*" I screamed.

Mom came running in the bathroom. I was standing there naked with my hands on my head horrified by the water.

"*Mags, Honey, look at me. Look at me!*" mom said, screaming.

I looked up and she was holding her hand out to me. I grabbed it and got in the shower. I had to have her hold my hand though. There was something bad about that water. I just couldn't figure out what.

White fluid started to come out of my nipples. It was awful. Why was there white stuff running down me as I showered?

I looked down again at my body. It was all distorted. There was a massive cut across my pelvic bone. What was that? Then it hit me again I had a baby. They cut that baby out of me. That baby was Allison. Where was she? Why couldn't I get to her? Why did my breasts hurt so much?

I felt weak, faint, confused, and sad. I then knew once again that yes I was a mother, I had a child, and my milk was drying up, and then remembered I had a C-section. Then to add to that my brain had gone far away.

Mom had explained that my milk would dry up. She said we were going to feed Allie with formula. I really didn't get what she was talking about. All I knew was that I didn't feel well at all.

This was just too much. I looked at my mom. Why did she keep having those slanty eyes? It was really getting on my nerves. I was holding onto her, still not trusting the water that was hitting my body. So many thoughts raced through my head as I tried to put some soap on myself as well as hold onto my mother.

Would I ever regain my old life? Would I ever be able to get back to Matt and love this new baby that had come out of me only less than a week ago. There was just too much to think about. As the warm water hit my body I felt like whatever I was able to give my newborn baby was now leaking out of me and drying up forever. I would never be able to feed her like a normal mother again.

The tears flowed down my cheeks. They felt hotter then the warm water hitting me. I felt empty, useless, and distraught. *Why couldn't I have something? Where was God? If He was there, why wasn't He healing me? Why, why, why ME?*

Breast-feeding was the one thing I could do and now I had to stop because of all the medications. "*PLEASE GOD WHY ARE YOU DOING TO THIS TO ME,*" I yelled aloud as the water continued to run down my empty body and mind.

My mom told me it would be okay. She said lots of moms had to use formula. I wasn't so sure about that. I got out of the shower and put on this tight sports bra she had bought for me. It was supposed to help dry up whatever was left. Gone, gone, gone.

I looked in the mirror. My reflection was awful. My eyes were glassy, my body slumped, my skin pale, there was no Maggie in there. Just a shell of my former self.

I wondered if I would ever come back. I felt dead. I was a useless mother that had lost her mind and had lost all contact with the outside world. I didn't know how to take care of a baby and I didn't care to learn. I didn't care about anything or anyone. I slowly put my stretched-out pale purple DKNY nightgown and slowly made my way a few steps to our tiny living room.

"Mom I want to hold Allison. Where is she?"

"Of course, Maggie", she stammered back.

She went into the office/nursery and out she came with my baby girl. She put her in my arms. I smiled for a moment at this cute little pink baby. Then I put her back in my mom's arms and walked over and picked up my guitar and started playing. It was like my brain remembered that I was a mother for just one brief moment in time and then, snap, it was gone again. My mom put my baby girl in my arms while she brushed out my wet hair. The baseball playoffs were on but I couldn't concentrate on them. I looked past the TV to a spot on the wall while my baby tried her best to get my attention. I gave her none and just concentrated on the spot. Then I gave my mom the baby back and went back to bed and rocked back and forth trying to get my brain back.

Out of the corner of my eye I saw in my journal a memory verse Carrie had written down for me. Another verse from the book of Philippians 3:13 "*Brothers and sisters, I do not consider myself yet to have taken hold of it. But one thing I do: Forgetting what is behind and straining toward what is ahead.*"

My mother had written a note next to it saying, "*Maggie, this means focus all your energy toward winning the race. Maggie, your race is Matt plus Allison plus all together plus wellness again.*" I read that again and again but still felt there was also one more thing missing but I couldn't put my finger on it.

Chapter 10

Home Life

That first week home was a trying time for my family. Matt was a physical education teacher and the field hockey coach for the girl's high school team. My mom was trying her best to keep me under control, reinforcing that I indeed was a mother, and teaching me how to take care of my new baby girl.

Matt's parents had gone home for some rest after all the intense problems with me. Before Matt's dad left he solved a massive problem. That was getting my medication. Nobody was able to get through to my psychiatrist. She was out of town and had left nobody else in charge of her patients to contact for medication refills. Luckily Matt's dad was a doctor and boy did that come in handy. He was able to get me back on my Depakote and contact a friend of his who was a psychiatrist. That doctor had suggested some medications that might help me bring me down a bit and get me sleeping.

My dad was constantly on the phone with me trying to reassure that I would be okay. My best friend Carrie called although I could focus for only a few minutes on what she was said. I was too out of it. My sister came over too, but again I didn't acknowledge her existence or love.

The days seemed to roll into one another. One minute it was morning and my mother had me holding the baby. Then there was always a nap time somewhere waiting around the corner.

Most of all there was the smell of diapers. It seemed like I was changing this baby every other minute or my mother was. It was so hard to keep trying to figure out what was real and what my head was making up.

My nights were the worst. By this time I was on some heavy medication so I could sleep through the night. The problem with this plan was the vivid nightmares, the kind where people's heads were coming off, the kind where blood gets spattered all over the room, the kind where everyone dies. I would wake up screaming, which as you can imagine would jolt Matt right out of bed in a flash. He would hold me until I would come to and then have me sit on the floor while he would change the sheets. My dreams where so awful I would soak right through the sheets.

He would also get a dry t-shirt for me to change into and new underwear. The medication got to be so intense Matt had to put me in Depends. I was so out of it I couldn't make it to the bathroom. Here I was 30 years old wetting the bed. Matt had not only a newborn's diapers to change but his wife's as well. He started doing this because dragging me to the toilet and trying to prop me on it wasn't working out too well. I would pee all over the sheets and the floor.

These were desperate times.

I knew this was taxing on Matt, but I couldn't help it. I was like a dead person. I was trapped in a prison of my mind unable to reach him. For maybe just a few moments in the middle of the night I remembered that Matt and I were new parents and we had a little baby. I could hear her little cry while Matt would soothe her and make her a fresh bottle. Then the next instant I would check right back out. Back I would go to the land of the darkest dreams I would ever face in my lifetime. He would stay up hours throughout the night feeding Allie and soothing her. His strength was his faith in Christ, which I would not find out until much later.

Chapter 11

Notes to the Family

I started leaving notes for my family and Matt's as well. I thought maybe it might be a better way to communicate with everyone since my brain was spinning too fast to tell them what I thought was vitally important information.

October 11, 2006

> ➢ Dr. Shaffer...

> ➢ Social Worker....be calm when she comes so she doesn't take my baby

> ➢ Mom is home...nobody else can come right now

- ➢ Give me eight hours to sleep so I can get better
- ➢ There is something wrong with these medications...I am getting worse
- ➢ Dad makes me hyper and mad
- ➢ Donna and Jim can only visit when I say
- ➢ Noises bother me, even phones ringing...make them stop, TV is driving me crazy, anyone talking irritates me
- ➢ The Paranoia is out of control...but I can't stop it.

I would write these notes in a Mead Composition notebook having only certain family members read it when I thought it was safe. It totally drove Matt, Mom, and everyone else nuts, but what could they do. I thought I could only truly communicate the vital information through this 99-cent book. I don't know how my family was able to be so patient during this trying time.

October 12th at 4:05am

I went to bed at 10:33pm. The drugs made me very tired. I had 2 Depakote, 1/4th clazonapam because it was needed. I also took a stool softener as well. I did not take any pain pills. My stomach does hurt though. I don't know why. I woke up at 2:05 with a throbbing toothache. I feel like it is killing me. I need you all to know how much pain I am in. There is something very wrong with me and this tooth thing. They are connected in some way and making me very sick. I think this tooth thing is making my manic stuff worse. My dreams tonight were the worst I have ever had. I woke up in a cold sweat from my mom shrieking at me. She wasn't though. It was only a dream but it seemed so real. I also dreamed of Donna yelling at me and I punched her in the face and blood went all over the walls. I cannot handle these awful dreams. They are very scary and too intense for me to handle. It almost seems my nights are worse than my hellish days I wake up too. I have tried to go back to sleep but I can't. I am now up for the day. Wondering how I will make it. I know I am very, very sick that is for sure but do not know how to get well. I thought by writing this down I might get better quicker.

I have written some goals down.

#1 ~ My brain (ha ha) is one side wants to answer all phone calls, e-mails, take long walks, and do lots of shopping

#2 ~The other side of my brain is urging me to slow down and get better, I want to not yell at my mom and dad, I don't want to cry anymore it wears me out, I want to get rid of the paranoia. How do I do this? I have bad sleep deprivation. This needs to be fixed. I will keep getting worse without sleep.

#3 ~ I will take my medication at the appropriate times. (Which truthfully I have done.)

Keep telling the truth. I hope Matt, mom, dad, and Carrie will keep believing me and Dr. S. too. I know I sound paranoid but I can't help it.

#4 ~ This is the most IMPORTANT GOAL

I want to be with our beautiful baby Allison and my husband again that I love so dearly AND get me well so I can achieve being normal again so I CAN HAVE MY FAMILY.

It is now 12 hours later in my notepad. It is 4:22pm to be exact. I don't like feeling manic like I did in 1996. This time I just want to be fixed. This is scary. I don't want to go back to another mental institution like I did ten years ago. I can't. I won't go. I can't be away from my baby and Matt. Please family don't take me away. It will only take me backward. I hate being irritated, delusional, ...enough said.

Oh another note for today we need to get this tooth fixed. I think I am having a bad reaction with the amphetamines that my body causes which again can cause me not to sleep plus have delusions. Get this fixed! Everyone needs to get on board. I can't fix this by myself.

October 13th ~ A Letter for Matt and Allie

Yes, maybe I did trick all of you the night I came home from the hospital. I guess I knew I was getting sick, but I thought I could manage this illness by myself.

I am very strong, family. You all must understand I am fighting like a mad to get back to you all. When we were at the pediatrician, I barely held it together. Thankfully Jim got me a snack out of the snack machine. I feel like if I am a little bit hungry I just lose all control and want to yell at people. I remembered today that Allison was born on a Monday October 3rd at 4:59. That was my mile goal time in high school! Looks like I got my wish but a baby girl. I will take it! I just need to know how to get better so I can be with her like normal moms do. How do I get well? Family, please figure this out. I am so sick.

To Matt and Allison, I love you both more than you could imagine. I will try to have patience today. I am trying so hard to get back to you both. Please don't give up on me. I will get better one day and we will get our life back

Love, Maggie and Mom

Chapter 12

Toothache

Not too long after we got home from the hospital my tooth started to kill. It was so bad my mother got me to a dentist right away that Matt's parents knew named Dr. Brassington. He knew I was very ill and was very calm and gentle with me. He made me feel relaxed. He looked in my mouth and said, *"Maggie, I am sorry to tell you this but you need a lot of work."*

It turned out I needed a root canal and I had nine cavities. The root canal was serious and needed to be dealt with right away.

Dr. Brassington gave my mom the number of a specialist that only did root canals and off we went. Matt stayed home with Allie while mom took me to my appointment in her bright yellow pickup truck.

For some reason my brain was set of by a siren that I heard in the distance. *"Mom, they are after us,"* I said.

"Maggie, I promise you nobody is after us," Mom retorted.

I just sat there in the truck in sheer terror. I felt like my heart was jumping out of my chest. The sweat was pouring off my body with such intensity my clothes became wet.

Only I knew who was coming and why. If only my mom would believe me. I scrunched down in the pickup as far as I could so they couldn't spot me.

Mom kept looking at me with those worried eyes again. Man, did that drive me nuts. I wanted to tear her eyes out.

Why couldn't she believe me? We were about to get captured. I could hear them coming. I was only trying to warn her about these awful people trying to get us. Just then I spotted them. They were helicopters and those helicopters were coming for our yellow pickup. I wished Mom had a four-door sedan. Then we could blend in with the rest of San Diego. But I knew we couldn't get away. Bright yellow was just too distinct. We were probably the only one in the entire city.

"I am hungry and thirsty Mom," I yelled suddenly.

Mom said, *"Maggie, I will try to find us a little something in a minute. We have a little time before the appointment. Please be patient while I look."*

Patience was not a word in my vocabulary. When I became hungry and thirsty, that needed to be taken care of right then and there. I started to count in my head to try to calm myself. I just needed that food, then I would be all right.

I wondered where we were going anyway? Oh wait, I know. It was to the dentist. Wait, why was I headed there again?

My head was spinning. The sounds were too intense. Why was everything so loud? Why did everything not make any sense? My head hurt. Everything hurt. My tooth started to throb. I needed food.

Finally we were pulling into the parking lot. There was a coffee shop of some sort in front of us. As we started to walk in I felt the eyes of everyone in the entire place on me. They all knew that those choppers were after us. My goodness it must be all over the news. Were there secret cameras on us? Must be.

"Mom, I need to sit down. Something is off. Way off," I stammered.

I slid down low in my seat and put my black hooded sweatshirt over my hair. Maybe people would stop looking at me if I could hide under some fabric.

Mom came back with a scone and a cup of tea. *"Maggie, this will help. It is really good and the tea will warm you up,"* she said.

I shoved the scone in my mouth and ate it as fast as I could. To others around me I am sure it was strange to see me shoving food in my mouth with crumbs falling everywhere and looking around everywhere all nervous and out of it. I drank the tea so fast I burned my tongue. It was like I forgot how to do all the basic functions. I had lost all ability to do the simplest of things and my paranoia was off the charts. On the way out I tried to cover my face the best I could which in reality only made me look more odd.

Back in the yellow pickup I felt the world watching us as we merged onto the freeway. There were many choppers following us now. I felt like I was in the movie *Goodfellas* when actor Ray Liotta has choppers following him at the end of the picture. It was absolutely terrifying. I told Mom this and she tried her best to convince me there was nothing.

As we pulled into the dentist office I was instantly on even higher alert. I ducked as I got out of the truck and quickly walked in. I went up to the lady at the check-in and yelled a couple of things at her.

My mom told me to go wait outside. What had just happened? I was so confused. I felt the woman was being rude to me so I told her so.

I was feeling a bit agitated now. My moods were switching increasingly fast which was making me tired.

I went back into the lobby, sank into a chair and closed my eyes. It felt like I hadn't had a full, restful night's sleep in months.

Just then Allie popped into my head. I was a mom. I had a little baby somewhere. I wondered where she was. "*Mom, where is Allie?*" I asked suddenly.

"*She is with Matt back at the house,* " mom said. "*I am glad you asked!*"

"Isn't she such a peanut...with those beautiful baby blues?" I said. But as I said this and looked at my mom I felt like I was losing her again. My brain flipped back off and whatever she was saying stopped registering in my head.

Just then the dental assistant came into the room and said, *"Maggie we are all ready for you."* I sat up straight at the call of my name.

"Go ahead," my mother said. I felt like a robot not a person. I awkwardly got to my feet and walked stiffly over to the lady, muttering under my breath. I couldn't remember where I was again. This was getting old.

The lady said, *"Hi Maggie, my name is Samantha. I am going to help the dentist today with your tooth."*

"Alright," I said. I lay down the best I could on a long, white, bed-like contraption. There were all kinds of tools around me. I thought they were going to torture me.

There were lights everywhere. Was that a gas mask? I was starting to panic.

Then some guy came over me and said he was the surgeon. Surgeon for what? I couldn't get the words out. So I started screaming for my mother, *"They are going to kill me!"*

The dentist and assistant were quite alarmed with my behavior. My mom came running in and I could hear her explaining that I was sick. She was right. Wasn't she? I was sick. Very sick. I needed to get better. I needed to get back to Matt and Allie. I wanted to be well again. With that I blacked out.

Chapter 13

Jackson Speaks

The next thing I knew I was back home. Where had I been the last 24 hours? I didn't know. I couldn't remember. Not a thing.

Then I heard a little cry. *"Mom, is that my baby I hear?"* I cried.

"Yes sweetheart," Mom said. *"I will go get her."*

I watched Mom get up. Where was she going? I was gone again.

I sat at my little kitchen table and looked around. It was so cute. I had painted this kitchen the prettiest color, sage green. It had the most beautiful little French doors going outside to our patio. It was a great space. This little house was heaven.

Jackson, my yellow lab, caught my attention. He was licking my feet and had his head tilted to the side. My mom walked in with something in her arms, but I paid no attention. I was listening to Jackson who was trying to tell me something. I thought he was trying to talk.

"*Maggie, here is Allie,*" Mom said.

I didn't hear her. I was only focused on the dog. "*Jackson, would you like a biscuit, boy,*" I excitedly said. "*I know you want a biscuit. You stay here. I will get you one.*"

I got up, got a bone and trotted over to Jackson. I gave him the bone and he answered, "*Thank you mommy.*"

Did my dog just talk to me! I think he did.

"*Mom,*" I yelled! "*Jackson is talking to me.*"

My mom had some tears on her face. Seriously why couldn't she be happy for my excitement! I mean, my dog was talking to me. I could get on Jay Leno with this dog! I could make millions.

"*Jackson, would you like to tell me something?*" I asked. He wagged his tail all crazy and was ready for more bones.

Next, I decided to have a tea party. "*Okay boy. We will have a bone tea party.*"

I set up some plates and put some toast on mine and a bone for his. I just started talking to him and I could hear all his thoughts. This was the most amazing day I had ever had. I mean who ever get to see their dog talk with them. It was something that only I had the power to see.

My mother didn't care. She was all wrapped in whatever she was holding. I wish there was somebody I could share my joy with. I will call Matt. He will understand. He will know what to do with a talking yellow lab. This will be our ticket to fame. Really, it will.

"Good boy, Jackson, you are such a lover dog," I said out loud.

I fed myself a bit then gave Jackson a little piece of his bone. He replied, *"Thank you."* I laughed and started all over again.

I picked up the phone to call Matt. All of the sudden I had this sinking feeling that he had died. I thought he was dead. Something bad had happened. I didn't know what, but he wasn't in the land of the living. I waited for the hum of the rings. One, two, three, four, rings went by. He wasn't answering the phone. He must be dead. Then a voice came on. It was Matt. I burst into tears.

"Maggie," the voice said. *"What is wrong honey? Is Allie alright?"*

I snapped back into reality for a few moments. I said, *"Matt, I thought you were dead. I thought you were not coming back. Jackson was talking to me. Nothing is making sense. I am tired."*

I could hear Matt talking, but couldn't focus on what he was saying. I gave the phone to my mom and ran to the back bedroom. I was very ill. I didn't know how to get well. I needed to write. I would write everything down so they would know how to get me better. I can't go on like this. I felt the effect of the medication making me groggy. Then I fell fast asleep.

Chapter 14

Making No Sense

My tooth felt better but my brain did not. I thought if my tooth was fixed my brain would clear. That was not the case. These were the medications the doctor prescribed for me so he could fix me, and my schedule.

> 7:00pm 1 Zyprexa
>
> 7:45-8:45pm Sleep
>
> 8:50pm 1/2 Zyprexa
>
> 9:45-10:30pm Sleep
>
> 10:45pm 1 Zyprexa
>
> 11:30-2:00am sleep
>
> 1/2 Zyprexa @ 2:30am
>
> SLEEP 3:00-5:15am

Matt was at work. My dad said Matt was safe, but I didn't believe him. I as very worried that he wasn't alright. I took more Depakote, Clonazepam and Ducolax at 7:45. I wanted to have a phone call to check on Matt. I needed to make sure he was alive. My two goals of the day were to take a shower and rest. I was exhausted.

Chapter 15

Dr. S

I had my journal with me. I was writing down everything so I could tell Dr. S how to get me well. My mother drove me to Del Mar. It was a quaint little beach down full of beautiful shops for the wealthy overlooking the sea. My doctor's office was just a block away from the ocean.

I had chosen Dr. S years ago because a friend of mine had told me about her. My friend Kimberly had gone to her for years and really liked her. She had told me about her office with the ocean view and the therapy dogs and what a cute town Del Mar was. Back then I thought -great combo. If you have to see a psychiatrist why not make it a fun place to go to. With golden retrievers and an ocean view. What is there not to like?

We had Allie with us in a purple baby carrier. She was so cute. I was feeling great today and knew I was a mother. I knew today I was going to get help and get back to my family.

"*Hi Theresa,*" I said as I floated in the door.

"*What a beautiful baby, Maggie,*" Theresa said in her thick Spanish accent. I could barely understand her.

Theresa and my mother started talking while I say down and looked down at my baby smiling. Maybe I would be better now and could be like all the other new moms out there. I was pretty happy. In fact very happy. My brain was clear.

Suddenly my reverie was interrupted by the screech of tires outside. I glanced out the window to see a well-dressed very pretty blonde in a red Mercedes convertible. She jumped over her door, raced up the steps and almost knocked my mother over.

"*Sorry,*" the woman said loudly. "*Hi Teresa, girlfriend. How are you? I am sorry I am late. I was just in a model shoot and got in a car wreck.*"

Theresa said, "*Oh, Taylor, sorry to hear that. I hate to tell you this but you have the wrong date for your appointment.*"

Taylor responded, "*Oh shit, really? Oh well. Hey you want to see my model pictures. I mean they just turned out fabulous.*"

Taylor looked at me. "*See I am a model. Do you want to see?*"

I didn't want to look at her dumb pictures. So I said, "*Look what I have? This is my new baby. Isn't she beautiful!*"

Theresa and my mom looked at each other not knowing exactly what to do with this exchange. Dr. S. came out of her office with a patient and was taken aback by all the talking and confusion.

Theresa said, "*Dr. S., Taylor came on the wrong day by mistake. I will reschedule her.*"

With a stern voice Dr. S. replied, *"Theresa, why don't you call her and do that later. We have way too many people in the office right now."*

Taylor piped in, *"Dr. S. look at my pictures!"* Jockeying for Dr. S's attention, I exclaimed, *"Well, look at my Allison!"*

After Taylor screeched back out of the small parking area in front I went on into the office while I heard my mother speaking in hushed tones to Dr. S. about my medications and my state of mind.

I was tired again and slumped down deep in the couch. I could hear the steady beat of the clock ticking. The room seemed different from when I last saw it. What was it? Oh, it was a different room. I had forgotten she had moved into a different room. She used to have an upstairs room with the ocean view. Now she was downstairs in a dark room. I didn't like it. I wanted light.

I immediately got up and opened up the shades. There that was better. I could think a bit better.

I gripped my black journal very tightly. I needed to get across all the recording I was doing in this journal today. It would be the way out of this sickness I had. I knew that I was in a manic episode and therefore that is why I was here in this very office today. We had a plan of action. We needed to get me back to my family. Back to the world or reality. Not the world of helicopters, death, and tea parties.

"Hello Maggie," Dr. S. said as she came in the door.

"Hi Dr. S," I replied as my eyes darted all over the room.

Dr. S started talking, but I didn't hear her. I was checked out. Her mouth was moving but I didn't hear a word she was saying.

I was trying to figure out where the recorder was. I bet she was taping this session. Maybe there was a hidden camera somewhere in this office. Was it by the big buffalo picture? Maybe it was by that clock that kept ticking way too loudly?

I started to feel like I needed to get out of there. I felt a sweat break out on my body. It felt as if my skin was crawling. I wanted out of my body. I wanted free from this prison I was in.

"*Maggie, how is your sleeping?*" asked Dr. S. Her voice brought me back and I realized I was being talked to.

I paused a while before I figured out how to form the words for the correct answer. "*I am having night terrors, I sleep on and off throughout the night, I sweat through the sheets,*" I stammered. I remembered my journal that my dad had given me to help to the doctor what I had been going through. Who knows if this would help, but I wanted to try everything I could think of to get better and fast.

"*When is my brain going to slow down?*" I said a little too loudly. "*I need to get back to my family! I need my life back!*"

My doctor calmly said, "*Maggie, it will all come back, with time. I am trying Seroquel on you with your Depakote. We will start on this lower dose and then work our way up. Plus, I want to get you sleeping better. I am going to put you on Ambien for sleep."*

All of this information was a lot to take in. The doctor wrote it all down, gave me prescription sheets, and some suggestions I might try to get through my days.

By the end of the hour I was so tired I felt like I just might pass out right then and there. I shuffled my feet as I left the doctor's office and looked slowly over at my mother holding Allie. I felt no connection with either of them. I just felt numb and wanted to lie down. I wanted to get to my bed.

My mom took care of scheduling the next appointment while I spaced out and thought of nothing.

Suddenly, just as if I had been hit by a storm, my brain switched into panic. I didn't know if Matt was alive or dead. Should I ask my mom? Should I ask Dr. S? Will they put me away if I tell them my thoughts? I decided I needed to keep the panic to myself. I would find out soon enough if Matt was alive when we got back home.

As my mother locked Allie's car seat into the backseat of the Jeep, I climbed as best I could and tried to figure out how to fasten my seat belt.

My mind was in a panic. My heart was beating too fast. I felt clammy and cold, and on the verge of death myself.

Mom jumped in the jeep said a few things that I couldn't make out. As we merged on the 5 freeway she accidentally hit the headlights off and couldn't turn them back on. "*Margaret, honey,*" she screamed. "*I don't know where the light switch is! Help!*"

Suddenly, like it was nothing to me, I reached my hand over and flipped the lights back on. Then, just like that, I went back into zombie mode. I could hear my mom saying something to me and being so thankful, but she seemed like a million miles away. I heard something behind me. Was that a baby cry? I don't know. I

slumped in my seat and fell fast asleep.

Maggie's Mom

The trip to Del Mar! That was a real winner! I met someone

sicker than Margaret - a red-letter day. Some part of me felt so

sorry for the girl who was a model though - I had a feeling she was

never going to get better - and I was getting confident that we were

improving. If you had asked me why I thought that, I don't know

what I would have said - just a feeling I guess.

Chapter 16

Dead in Africa

Later I awoke to my mother talking on the phone to Donna.

I could hear my mother talking about Matt's brother Todd, his wife

Laura, and their baby girl, Cami, who was about a year and a half

old. All I heard was that they were sick with malaria, and from that,

I believed that they had all died. Worse yet, my mother was trying

to keep this from me. I was sure of it. She was just making up that

malaria stuff so I wouldn't freak out.

Todd, Laura, and their little girl were in Togo, Africa. I

never was happy about them going there. They were doing

missionary work there. To me, it seemed that Togo was a scary place full of disease, dishonest people and an unstable government. So I figured some bad people must have come in their compound and killed them.

I thought about that I had the power to bring Todd's family back. If I could pray to God enough, non-stop, they would come back to life. I knew I could make this happen. So I started to pray out loud, crying plaintively as I did so.

Hearing this, my mom ran in the bedroom, concerned with my behavior. "*Margaret, what is going on,*" she said all flustered.

"*Don't worry, Mom,*" I cried. "*I can bring them all back from the dead. I know they died in Togo. It is alright though I can do this. It is in my powers from God.*"

I started to hyperventilate from my heavy breathing. My mom ran to the kitchen and returned with a paper bag.

"*Maggie, you must believe me,*" she yelled so I would look at her.

"*They are all fine, just a bit sick from Malaria.*"

I didn't hear this though. I jumped under the covers and screamed for God to bring them back from the dead.

I could hear my mom on the phone to my doctor. I started to scream. Mom came running back in.

"*Mom, they are not going to make it,*" I yelled frantically.

My mom figured there was no sense in trying to talk me out of my frantic state so she said, "*Maggie, pray away, and get back under the covers if you think that helps.*"

I did as I was told and yelled out prayers under the sheet. Jackson jumped on the bed next to me. I grabbed onto him, held him tightly and cried. I was losing my family somewhere in Africa and there was nothing I could do about it.

I looked frantically for my Mead pad where I had written more Bible verses Carrie had given me. I found James 1: 2-5. It read, "*Consider it pure joy, my brothers and sisters whenever you face trials of many kinds, because you know that the testing of your faith produces perseverance. Let perseverance finish its work so that you may be mature and complete, not lacking anything. If any of you lacks wisdom, you should ask God, who gives generously to all with finding fault, and it will given to you.*"

The words slowly sank into my head for a few minutes. I felt some peace come over me as I laid my head on Jackson's belly and fell fast asleep.

Later I came to only to realize none of what I thought had happened. My brother-law and my niece were sick with Malaria but not dying. Everything was going to be all right at least for the moment anyway.

I felt so worn out from the screaming and crying fit that I could hardly lift my head. Jackson was still lying on the bed with me. He looked at me and gave me a big lick on the face. I fell back against him and was so confused by my actions. Why had I thought I had powers? Why was it so real that my relatives had died? These were questions I couldn't answer. I needed to talk to Matt.

"*Mom*," I yelled. "*I need to talk to Matt. I need to check and make sure he is alright.*"

Our day went on like this for endless hours. I would check in and know everyone was living and then the next moment think that again my relatives were dying somewhere in the continent of Africa.

The only saving grace for that day was every now and then picking up my journal and reading the verses from James 1: 2-5. Something deep inside my core was starting to shift.

Chapter 17

Screw You!

I woke up and I couldn't quite understand what was happening. I felt as if I was in some weird dream. In University Heights we all lived practically on top of each other so I could hear every little thing that happened next door. I heard yelling, banging around, and some loud crazy person yelling *"Screw You."*

It was still dark so I decided it was better if I tried to go back to sleep. Only I couldn't. My mind was racing once again and I had to figure out what the hell was happening next door.

I felt Matt next to me, sleeping soundly. How could he do that? He was in a perfect place of peace. Oh how I wished I could have his body for one day. One day of freaking peace.

I heard a faint sound from the other room. It was like a little whimper.

Unreal! I had forgotten once again I had a baby in the next room. This made me feel like absolute shit. *"Why am I so nuts? Why can't I be like all the other moms out there and be thrilled I have a baby in the next room?"*

I was not thrilled though. I was horrified. I was afraid because I didn't know how to be a mom. I didn't know the first thing about taking care of a child. I didn't even want to get up and check on her. Again this made me feel more depressed.

My body hurt. I felt the stitches on my lower abdomen. Yes, this was where the baby came out. Yes, I had a C-section. That baby has a name and it is Allison. I need to love her.

As my mind kept trying to figure out the baby situation I heard more cussing.

"*Screw you! Screw you!! Screw You!!!*" Then I heard dead silence and more banging around.

Matt mumbled in his sleep about Leanne and her crazy drug brother making all the noise and then back to sleep he went.

I heard the yelling start again This time it went on without stopped and at a higher volume. "*What is going on! I can't take this anymore.*"

I opened the window and yelled at the top of my lungs at the neighbors who were no more than five feet away.

"*SHUT the hell up! I can't take all this racket. If you don't shut up I am calling the cops!*"

All I heard was more rustling around and then a strange squawking sound. Did Leanne have a parrot in there? Who knew? Matt said she was a hoarder. There was so much stuff in her house it went from floor to ceiling and it was like a mini maze to get from one room to another. What ever was going on over there was bad. I knew that much.

At the house, I would see Leanne's brother, Avery, and his druggy friends come and go at all times of the day and night. I decided I might feel better if I got up and went to the bathroom. I felt terribly sick from all the medications my doctor was pumping through me. I felt wet as I stumbled to our cute little bathroom, I realized I must have peed in my pants in the middle of the night. Really? 31 years old I couldn't even make it to the bathroom because I was so out of it on medication that I couldn't wake up.

I started a bath because I was so grossed out. The warm water felt good on my torn-up post-pregnancy body. I didn't think I was supposed to sit in a bath because of these stitches but at this point I couldn't care less. I needed to feel good for one moment. The bath seemed to do just that.

I decide to pour an entire bottle of shampoo in the tub so I could have a crazy bubble bath and not have to look at my distorted body. I wanted to imagine I was at the Ritz Carlton soaking in the perfect bathtub, getting ready for some awesome party.

When I lived in San Francisco I lived at the corner of Powel and California in a hostel-like apartment building. I had my own studio but shared a bathroom with 4 other people who lived close to me. The Ritz Carlton was two blocks down from my building and I would wander down there from time to time and walk through the hotel pretending to be a guest. Sometimes I would sit in the lobby and have a drink. As I would sit there, I would imagine what it would be like if I was truly a guest there. I would take a long bubble bath with a glass of ice tea and then dress in the most beautiful white outfit from Nieman Marcus, and amazing shoes of course.

It was hard to believe that now, 10 years later, I was married, had a baby in the next room, and had just closed my mini day spa business. Would I ever have my own life and have fun again?

Was it extremely selfish to feel this way? Well, yes, it was. I sank deeper into the bubbles ashamed of my thoughts.

In the distance I heard the crackling sound of my neighbors fighting yet again, "Screw you, Screw you, Screw you."

I sank under the water so I couldn't hear those mean words. They reminded me of my sick days when I became manic at 19, spent time institutionalized at Stanford Medical Center, and was diagnosed with Bipolar Disorder I, the most severe kind there is.

Yet here I was at 30 years of age, once again manic, out of my mind, and terribly ill once again. I couldn't seem to connect with my baby or my husband, or anyone for that matter.

Part Two:
Limping Along
On
Three Cylinders

Chapter 18

Side Effects

The medication that I was on were intense. I was on

Depakote, Seroquel, Ambien, and Abilify and possibly others

because I was blindly taking what was given to me. The side effects

were intense. First of all I was starving all the time. Even though I

ate more than enough food I was still hungry. My mom tried her

best to keep me away from the refrigerator. In one day I ate ten

mini burgers plus snacks and I was gaining weight rapidly. I wasn't

really aware of this, but everyone else could see what was

happening and tried their best to help.

I didn't know which reaction came from which medication either. My mind was so tired, so fast, and worn out. My hands trembled, my right leg was shaking non-stop, and my eyes were glazed over.

I knew my family was out there. I knew I needed to get better so I could get back to them. I knew I had a baby but I didn't know how to reach her. I was trapped in my sick, broken-down body and mind.

Even though I was so out of it, with all the medication my mom would have me dressed and ready to take baby Allie on a walk twice a day. It would take us about hour to get going and then another hour to get to the park, which was only a couple blocks away.

I moved so slowly. Pushing my purple stroller along the cracked sidewalks of the community of University Heights right by downtown San Diego. I would run into one of the cracks and stop not knowing that I needed to lift the wheels up a bit to get going again. My mother would help get me going again and talk about Allie. I didn't really listen to anything she said and didn't really care that I was pushing whatever was inside the stroller. I was so gone I was numb. My body hurt all over and I couldn't figure out what was happening from moment to moment. It was awful. It was a hell I had been in once at 19 but this was worse. I knew I had a husband, a new baby, a house, and a life to get back too. But I couldn't. I had fallen into an abyss that was too deep to crawl out of.

When we would reach Trolley Barn Park it was always a strange feeling that would come over me. Mom would have me stroll over to where moms were talking about their children or new babies they were holding.

"See Maggie, soon you can meet some new moms here!"

What the hell was she talking about? I wasn't going to come hang out with people and their babies.

I slowly strolled pass this group daily contemplating this new world that I had never noticed before nor ever wanted to know. I just wanted my old life back and wanted to think with a clear head. All this baby talk was too much.

I would always do the same loop with mom everyday with my legs feeling like they were full of lead. The medications were just too hard on my body and my mind. I didn't feel as if they were helping me at all. It actually felt like the combination of all the drugs just made everything worse.

With my mind going at warp speed, but my body moving like a snail, we would finish our loop and head back to my small bungalow on Louisiana Street. It wasn't so long ago that Matt and I would take our lab Jackson for a walk through these adorable little streets, eat at the bistros, have a glass of wine, and walk home hand in hand laughing without a care in the world.

That life was gone and this new life was here. I didn't know how to adjust, I didn't know how to be a mother, a wife, and these medications were killing me. I could feel my mood doing a major downshift.

I was starting to absorb how devastating things were. I couldn't communicate with my baby, with Matt, with anyone.

I needed something but what? I was an empty shell. I needed peace. Why couldn't God heal me like Carrie had said? Why was I under this attack? God please take this away I whispered to nobody.

I picked up my phone and called Carrie again. She said I needed to read Romans.

"Carrie I can't. God doesn't help me. I am so done," I cried.

"*Maggie, you are not done. Stop talking like that,*" she said. "*I am going to read you Romans Chapter 5 verses 3-5. All you have to do is listen.*"

I wrote it down in my journal so I could reference this for later. I was desperate. Romans 5:3-5 read, "*Not only so, but we also glory in our sufferings, because we know that suffering produces perseverance; perseverance character; and character, hope. And hope does not put us to shame, because God's love has been poured out into our hearts through the Holy Spirit, who has been given to us. (NIV)*"

The verse couldn't have been more perfect for that very moment. Once again I was filled with hope for that day. Maybe someday I would be made whole again.

Before she hung up Carrie prayed for me and I just took it in not knowing Jesus was starting to open my stubborn heart a little at a time. I scribbled in my journal, Believe day after day that

this can happen.

Chapter 19

"For We live by FAITH, not by Sight"

My dad came to visit for a few days and help my mom out.

He could tell I was pretty badly off. With checking on Matt

throughout the day to make sure he was alive, to talking nonsense,

it was very evident I was a long way from emerging from the

clutches of madness. My mother was really tired of driving me up

to Del Mar to my Psychiatrist, so my dad took over doing the 30-45

minute drive each way.

On one trip, we were there a little bit early. I was very

anxious and my mind started to race like crazy.

"Mags, lets go down and eat something. I saw a little soup and salad place. Getting something in your tummy will help you," he says.

I couldn't get out any words so I just follow his lead and we headed for the small eatery down the block. We got a table off to the side.

"Dad," I whispered. *"I think Matt just died."* My eyes are completely empty as I say this. I look like an empty shell.

"Listen to me Margaret!" Dad says. *"He is fine Honey. You must believe me. I can go call him if you would like."*

I don't hear him though. I am deep in my thoughts of death. I picture Matt lifeless with his eyes rolled back in his head. There is no life. Just a bloated dead body that was once my husband. Dad sees that he has lost me to my demented brain. He leaves a 20 on the table and takes me by the hand. We keep walking until we are at the beach. I feel myself in such a panic that I start screaming. My father just holds me until I almost pass out. It is too much for any father to bear.

"Margaret, you must believe that you will get well. God is there for you. He will heal you. Be patient Margaret, He has not forgotten you. He loves you. Believe me Margaret!"

He grabs me tight as he says this. My tears are rolling down my cheeks.

"Dad, if God is there why am I being tortured? Why is this happening to me again? I can't take my mind going away again! I want my life back dad. I want Allie and Matt back," I screamed.

We just sat there on the beach holding each other while I screamed and cried to the wind. After what seemed like an eternity, I started to calm down and Dad turned to me and said, *"Margaret, do you remember the very first memory verse your brother learned and said it until we were blue in the face?"*

"*Yes,*" I said with a sob.

Dad quoted 2 Corinthians 5:7 "*For we live by faith, not by sight.(NIV) That is what you need to hold onto Margaret your faith in God.*"

"*I don't have any, Dad,*" I cried.

"*Yes you do Margaret,*" Dad cried softly. "*You just don't remember. He has been with you this entire journey Margaret. Sometimes we don't know why we go through such pain but only HE will end our sadness. Give your worry to Him.*"

I leaned into dad and just let out deep wrenching sobs I didn't even know I could make. I could feel Dad's tears landing on me too which made it all the worse. How could I get this faith in God that my dad had? All I could see was pain all around me.

"*Maggie, listen. God doesn't give us more than we can handle,*" Dad said softly.

"*Okay Dad, let's go,*" was all I could muster.

Chapter 20

It Takes a Village

My mother was on watch 24/7 for the first month. She had

taken me to every psychiatrist, dentist, and pediatrician

appointment. The errands were endless and don't forget she was

not only taking care of me but of my new baby girl Allie. Ten

diapers per day, the naps, changing her clothes, boiling the bottles,

and feeding her! Between all of that, she was trying to get me to lie

down, tell me that Matt was not dead, draw charts that I could

check to see when I could call Matt to see if he really was living, and

trying to keep me from eating the entire house in a day.

It was just too much. It would be for anyone not matter how strong they were. She had Matt's mom Donna come in for a couple weeks of relief. I didn't want my mother to leave me and begged her to stay. I was unsure of having Donna help me. I didn't like that I was so ill and didn't want her to be in my presence. It wasn't that I was trying to be mean. I was just so ill. I didn't want anyone but my mother and Matt.

My mom had to have rest and so she went and Donna came much to my dismay. She did an amazing job. She was patient when I was unkind. She took care of Allie with the kindness of a Saint, and went above and beyond what was expected. I showed no love toward her, no gratitude, just felt angry. The good thing was it made me want to start trying to be a mother.

Something in my brain switched on that week and I really started trying to learn what was expected of me a new mother. I really tried to feed Allie rather than having my mother-in-law do everything. Donna kept me beside her, helping me get my hands wet being a new mom. There was a lot of trying moments that in those weeks but Donna made it work. She took it with great stride and just poured love on our family. I had her write in my little Mead Composition book as well so we all might find help and progress through everyone's thoughts toward me getting well.

I wrote notes next to the verse for her so she could better understand which she also really liked a lot. I summarized that you have been through some difficult times, but God will restore you to health!

My mom and Donna did their best to hold down the fort while Matt worked at his high school job. Everyone was drained. There were no breaks, and throughout the day everyone's mood would be bleak. It was hard to keep looking to the positives when I would continually ask if Matt was dead or if others had died that I knew. My reality was gone.

We needed extra help besides just the family but who and where? My mother had been asking around her church and friends up north if they knew of anyone that could possibly help our situation. A friend of hers from her church had an idea and my mom loved it. She called up Donna and presented her plan over the phone. She wanted Donna to interview Doulas. A Doula is someone that is like a Nanny but does much more. A Doula is woman that comes in usually for the first week for a new mother and helps them get going and learn the ropes.

Mom and Donna thought it would be a positive environment for someone else to help me be a mom rather than my mom telling me what to do and my mother-in-law. So that week we had two different interviews. I had no connection to the first lady that came and the idea was seeming hopeless until Anne arrived. When she came in I felt calm and knew immediately I needed this lady to teach me how to be a good mommy. I sat curled up in my sweatpants in Matt's old leather chair quite in peace as she talked.

She was from Belgium and her thick accent relaxed me. So the plan

was that she would arrive everyday at 8 and leave at around 2 just

as Matt got home from work.

Monday 10/23/06 Donna Reese

Enjoyed a neighborhood walk, It was just Allie, Maggie, Jackson, and me. Mag wants to see family tonight. She wisely doesn't want to go to a restaurant but has asked if we could just meet at Bill and Clarice's home. We are house-sitting for them in Point Loma. Mag has taken 1/4 Cloznepam, which is her ideal so she could stay focused and continue a great afternoon.

Praises to Mag ~

She initiates baby mommy time 3x this afternoon and evening

She recognizes living room is hot and fixes it by turning on ceiling fan, opening windows for cross breeze, and she went to garage and got out the portable fan. (Great problem solving)

She is initiating taking a shower and is able to dress herself (good organization)

We went off to Bill and Clariece's for the Reese family dinner. There was great interaction with Matt's cousins Vanessa, Kristen. Also with them 6 month old Ethan, Aunt Pat, Aunt Jan and Uncle John as well as Jim and me. It was a very pleasant and relaxed evening without any bad episodes. It was our best day yet. A real Victory for healing. If tomorrow dips, be encouraging. We are on the healing track!

I have noticed when she has anxiety and paranoia, prayers and hugs help. I wrote down a Bible verse, which she really liked.

Psalm 71 :19-21 *"Your righteousness, God reaches to the heavens, you who have done great things. Who is like you, God? Though you have made me see troubles, many and bitter, you will restore my life again; from the depths of the earth you will again bring me up. You will increase my honor and comfort me once more. (NIV)"*

Chapter 21

Anne

I woke up the next day looking forward to learning about this new Anne lady my mom and Donna had hired. Would it be a disaster or quite the opposite?

I put on my clothes, brushed my teeth, and actually cared a little what I looked like, as I got ready for the day. I even remembered I had little baby Allie in the nursery. Maybe something in my brain was starting to shift and just maybe I would get a little taste of what it might be like to have my old self back but blended in with a child.

I peeked out the white sheer curtains of our tiny home and watched Anne gathering her things. Matt was already outside giving some last minute instructions before he drove off to work in his silver Mustang convertible. I wonder if I will ever ride in that car again? It wasn't so long ago that I was driving his car around with the top down blaring Madonna's latest hit "Hung Up". Now, two months later I was a distorted shell of a woman who had lost her brain and couldn't remember I had a baby half the time. It was just like some alien had taken over my body and didn't care for the most part that I had a baby or a husband.

It was just crazy that I was like this. Why couldn't I get a handle on this? I knew I was sick but with all the medication the doctor was giving me why couldn't I just snap out of this fog and love my baby girl and connect with my husband. They were so far away. It seemed like an ocean was between us. My heart was empty.

I heard the doorbell ring. Since I could reach the door from my chair I didn't have to run to get the door. I just threw my leg over it and opened it.

"*Hi Maggie,*" Anne said. "*It is good to see you again. I am really looking forward to working with you!*"

"*Yes. Hi Anne. Matt said you would be here early. Looks like nobody trusts me being a mother so that is why you are here. Did you know I have Bipolar? Did you know I have it really bad? I forget about what is going on just about every other second. Are you here to be my nurse? If you are you might as well leave. I don't need a nurse. I really just want my old life back but everyone says I need to adjust. I don't get it. I am taking all my medications, taking care of the baby, cleaning, and trying my best to please Matt. What am I supposed to do? Oh yeah, my mom wants me not to drive while I am on medications. How is that going to work? I can barely make it to the mailbox without feeling like I might just pass out.*"

All of a sudden, I realized I was talking non-stop. There was no pause in my talking. It was like how a child starts to talk about something and they can't stop themselves.

I was immediately embarrassed by my actions and lack of control. I hadn't even mentioned Allie and where her room was.

The guilt closed over me like a black, dark cloud. I had this beautiful baby and hardly knew she was there unless someone else asked. How could anybody be this soulless? I guess it was me.

Why was I not bonding with this child? My thoughts were so fast I could keep up with them. I excused myself and ran into the bathroom to collect my thoughts.

The black and white checkered floors in the bathroom seemed dirty to me. I immediately had the urge to clean the bathroom. Just as I was about to go get cleaning supplies I heard a baby cooing and Anne talking softly. Right, I have a baby and Anne here. The cleaning will have to wait.

I took two steps right and I was in the nursery/office. There was Anne holding little Allison Isabelle in a cute little cow print blanket that was given to us by my mom's good friend Debra. Wow! I could remember who gave us what, but not that I was a mother every other second.

I could feel a tear trying to squeeze itself out and slide out of the corner of my eye. This was just too much. I needed to go lie down. All of a sudden I was felt overcome by exhaustion. *"Anne, do you mind if I lie down while you hold Allison? I need to rest a second."*

I took a couple of steps across our miniature house and I was already lying down on my big burgundy wine velvet couch. I thought I feel asleep but in reality I was there for about a minute and then jumped up and was running over to where Anne was with Allie again.

"Maggie, it would be good for you to rest longer," Anne said kindly. Her Belgian accent soothed me. I didn't argue, as I would have with my mother, but did what she said and tried to lie back down.

My mind was going so fast. It felt like the room was spinning. I could hear the clock ticking way too loudly and it was in the kitchen.

I hated this feeling of my life being out of control. I couldn't grasp simple concepts. Thank heavens my mom and mother-in-law hired Anne. There was no way I could care for my baby being this out of it. I didn't know how to feed her, bathe her, change diapers, and even how to hold her!

As my mind sped from thought to thought I could hear Anne carrying Allison around, talking to her as she did the feeding and changing. Maybe I could learn this mother stuff. Maybe Anne would teach me how to be a good mom and a caring one.

My heart was beating too fast. The anxiety was welling up again. I tried to breathe calmly. I just needed to get through this day. I shut my eyes super tight hoping it was all a bad nightmare. It seemed every breath I took was killing me slowly.

Just then I could hear Anne calling to me. *"Maggie, why don't you come to the nursery and I will teach you how to swaddle Allison,"* she said in her singsong voice. Again she put me into a calm trance as I made my way to trying out the first step to being a mother.

"Just put the blanket like this, curve this edge and that one," she instructed. I tried doing what she suggested as best I could and then laid Allison down in the center of the blanket. Little by little I made my first attempt at swaddling little Allie.

I found myself looking forward to my time with Anne every day. I would be waiting at the door 10 minutes before she would even show. I would pace back and forth with much anticipation until her car would pull up. Immediately I would sense some relief

as she would open up our small gate and walk up to the house.

"*Hi Anne*," I said with much excitement. "*Look what I did!*"

I motioned her to Allie's room where I had already dressed her for

the day and had her swaddled in her blanket.

"*Maggie, I am so proud of you*," Anne said. "*You are doing a

fantastic job.*"

Just hearing this encouragement made my mood soar.

Maybe there was hope after all. Maybe I would make a great

mother.

Anne started me on a routine daily that not only helped me

learn to be a good mom but also helped me start to gain my brain

back piece by piece. Every time my mind would start to wonder off

track she would gently pull me back in. She would tell me about her

family in the Netherlands or the sand dollars she would collect at the beach by her home. This would snap me out of my state and I would collect my thoughts so I could listen.

Anne got me over to the park everyday. She taught me about what I should pack in Allie's little diaper bag and put in the stroller. On our walks, Anne would point out how Allie was singing or playing with the little toys we hung on the stroller.

"Look how Allie is singing herself to sleep," Anne said. I looked down at my little peanut and sure enough she was cooing herself to sleep. I think I was starting to love this little being. She was growing on me and my brain was starting to give me a small break.

Anne was also awesome in teaching me about what to do on our outings to the store. Just coaxing me to park maybe a little farther away from others was such a good idea. Then I wasn't nervous about cars being to close to us. Getting out the stroller could be done without being stressed if others were trying to get by.

Taking my time made things easier. It was a huge process. I had to set up the stroller, put the brake on, get Allie out of her car seat, click that to the stroller, and then put the diaper bag on the end of the stroller. That is a lot to remember when your brain is going really fast.

If I didn't have Anne helping me remember all the steps I never would have made it into the store. This may sound awful, but without Anne I might have left my child in the car!

Chapter 22

Our First Road Trip ~ Tahoe Christmas

I had no idea how much planning I had to do to go on our first road trip with our new baby girl! Anne again was such a huge help here. We got out the suitcase a week before the trip and everyday would start preparing for what we would need.

Since we were headed to South Lake Tahoe to see Matt's parents I needed to pack for cold weather. Anne taught me all about having layers for Allie. We packed all kinds of outfits, socks, diapers, and warm outerwear. Then we prepared all the formula, bottles that we would need, bibs, a travel crib, and more endless supplies.

I don't even know how a sane person could do this job by themselves! We also packed my bag early so I didn't need to worry about that too.

I could tell Matt was very excited to go on this trip. He had been through so much with me since Allie was born. I so badly wanted to be well for him. I wanted that connection back that we had always had.

I could see that worry in his face and I would space out when he talked to me every night. I wanted to hear what he was saying or watch the football game with him but my mind would just drift.

"Maggie, did you just hear what I said?" he would ask.

"Sure, sure, I heard you. I just can't figure out what you are trying to tell me," I responded. It was tough for both of us.

That week went fast and before I knew it we were off in our Jeep Cherokee driving down the 5 freeway for first big road trip with a baby. Every inch of the Jeep was packed full of baby stuff. I sat next to Allie in the back seat, constantly playing with her pacifier and flicking her little toys to keep her entertained.

Matt drove with our favorite Jack Johnson music on while our 100 pound yellow lab took up a large portion of the back along with the luggage. It took us 10 hours to get to my parents' house when it usually takes about 7 1/2 hours. I think we stopped every 2 hours to change diapers and feed Allie.

The trip was quite a process, but we made it. I was pretty worn out, as was Matt, when we reached my parents. Everyone was overjoyed to see us, and especially Allie.

There was never a dull moment with having a new baby to show off. I wished I could enjoy everyone's excitement but I was so off. I felt distant and disconnected. It was as if I was hardly there and instead was watching my family from a distance. My mom made us one of her big ranch dinners, which tasted so good and I was able to sleep that night without the awful nightmares I had been having at home.

The next morning we left for the last leg of our trip to the mountains. Matt's parents had bought a vacation home there which had been such a fun place for all of us to meet up. I was very nervous about being around Matt's mom. I am not sure why I felt like this, but that's the way it was. I was not confident in my mothering skills and didn't want it to show. As we dropped into the Lake Tahoe area my worries subsided. There was so much beauty all around us. A soft snow blanketed the landscape, covering all the trees. Such a beautiful sight.

Matt's parents, Jim and Donna, were very happy about our safe arrival. From the moment we arrived, Jim and Donna showered us with their help. Donna wanted to help so much that my worries began to disappear. She changed Allie, helped with the feeding, and made me feel comfortable. I set up Allie's clothes, crib, and bottles. Even thought I was pretty checked out from what was going around me, I was able to enjoy life around me for the first time in a very long time.

Jim wanted to go out and search for a Christmas tree the next day. I strapped Allie to my front in a pack and off we went on our first little adventure together in the snow. The neighbor Judy came up with us too, which added to the enjoyment. I had gotten to know her very well over the past years.

"I think Maggie should choose the tree," Judy said. I found the tree I thought was best and everyone agreed that it was the perfect Christmas tree. Matt and his dad cut the pine tree down and hauled it back while Judy, Donna, Allie, and I took our time, taking in the snowy surroundings. That evening we decorated the

tree and put up some lights. Now this was starting to feel like Christmas!

Matt very much wanted me to go out snowboarding with him the next morning. I was extremely anxious about whether I would be able to this, but I wanted so badly to please him that I agreed to go. My heart was racing as I left Allie with Donna and headed to Heavenly Ski Resort. Was it because I was leaving my baby for the day or was I scared of snowboarding? I think it was both. Inside it felt like I was having a heart attack. I was sweating profusely inside my ski clothes and felt the urge to run. I kept my composure as best I could.

"Mag, don't worry," Matt said. *"You have done this for 15 years."*

"I know Matt," I said. *"But I feel like I am going to fall off the lift. I don't know if I can do it."*

As Jim dropped us off I could feel his worry about us too. In that moment, I felt that his worry was for his son and not me. He wanted Matt to enjoy himself and not be stressed. I could understand that; everyday Matt was dealing with a very sick wife.

"Enjoy today Matt and Maggie. I know you can do this," he said with a tear running down his cheek.

As we got on the Gondola my stress only intensified as we went up to the top of the mountain. I envisioned the Gondola falling off the cable and us crashing down the mountain with blood all over. I tried very hard to breath in and out and block those awful visions that were always trying to take over my consciousness.

I thought of baby Allie and began to calm down. I knew she was in good hands and that made me feel at peace. By the time I got off the lift I was able to strap my boots to the board and slowly make my way down the mountain. With all the medication and my mind racing it was hard to gauge my speed. I wasn't the confident

boarder I had been, but at least I was out there. Matt was very

patient, waiting for me at the bottom of each run. Usually I

boarded right behind him so this slower, more hesitant Maggie was

definitely out of the ordinary for us. By the end of the day I was

very tired, but glad I had agreed to go. Snowboarding together was

a part of pre-baby life that we were a step closer to recapturing, and

the day had brought Matt and me a little closer together.

Our week in Tahoe went by fast and there wasn't too much

stress. All the assistance and company helped me mentally. We

spent the next week at my parents. It was fun to see old friends but

also hard. The tough part was trying to figure out what was going

on some of the time. It took a lot of focus on my part to understand

what people were telling me. Even though my brain had slowed a

little it was still difficult to follow conversations. I am not sure

people knew how bad I was feeling since on the outside I looked fine. That is definitely a very strange aspect of mania. You look fine on the outside but are a disaster on the inside!

My good friend Mandi came by to meet Allie one of the days while we were at the ranch. It was so stressful trying to not act all crazy. My goodness, the last thing I wanted was to have my childhood friend see how sick I was.

My eyes were glazed over by all the medications I was on and my leg was still having the shakes worse than usual. I put Allison in my arms and decided to sit on the rocking chair awaiting her arrival. I am sure I was quite a sight sitting there all dazed out rocking away but she never let on that she knew something was wrong. She brought her two sons that I just adored as well. Ethan and Tyler were so awesome with baby Allie, which began to make me feel at ease.

"Maggie, you are doing a great job," Mandi offered. *"I know its draining in the beginning but you will get the hang of it in no time,"* she said in a very encouraging voice.

"I hope so," I said with my voice a bit slurred.

It was really nice to be with my parents for Christmas as well, but I could feel the depression weighing me down from deep inside. It felt like somebody was suffocating me.

The nights were always the toughest. From all the vivid nightmares of Allie dying to me jumping of a cliff, to watching others that I knew and cared for die, I was a wreck. I felt no relief by the time I would wake up in the morning. The sheets would be soaked. Sometimes it was so bad Matt would change them in the middle of the night.

At least at my parents' home I felt so comfortable, was fed my mother's good food, and didn't have to put on an act for them.

I could just be me, and knew I was not expected to make everyone around me feel comfortable.

If I was silent they would just let me be. Mom would just put on some good music and take care of Allie.

It was like watching a reality show that I was not a part of. Everyone was talking about all kinds of interesting topics, enjoying the Christmas atmosphere, and eating all the good food. I tried my best to participate, but it was rough.

In the evening my dad came home from the feed store that he had been running for over 40 years. *"Margaret, I know it is not looking good, but great days are ahead,"* he told me. *"You know I'm always right, don't you!"*

"Yes, Dad," I replied. *"It just seems so far away, you know. Being happy and feeling that love for my child, and that pride of being a mom doesn't feel like it is anywhere in sight."*

"Well, you know what, Margaret?" he asked.

"What Dad?" I said weakly.

"The good Lord won't let you down Mags. He never does."

"I feel like I have been let down, Dad," I said. *"Seriously, who gets this crazily sick in the head after having a baby? I am a paranoid freak most days with hardly enough brain cells to get through each day."*

"Dad, I feel like I am dying a little bit every day. My old life is completely gone, I am on so many medications I have become a lunatic just from the stupid side effects, and I feel like Allie is sucking the very life out of me," I stammered, on the verge of tears.

"Margaret, you must give God time," my dad said. *"He will heal you as good as new. Just believe in Him. Never doubt Him! Carrie left you a bible verse I am supposed to give you,"* he said. *"It is Psalm 8:9: 'Lord, our Lord, how majestic is your name in all the earth!"* (NIV)

"Right, Dad!" I cried. *"I am done with this bullshit!"*

I didn't mean to cuss but I was now upset and sad all at once. I didn't believe all this God stuff my dad kept telling me. He had been feeding me this since I first went psycho after bringing Allie home from the hospital. Dad hugged me and I cried harder than my baby crying upstairs.

Chapter 23

Sex Again? ~ Seriously, Just Shoot Me Already

Matt wanted to have sex again, which for me was the furthest thing from my mind. With the C-section, my mania, postpartum depression, and having gained all the weight from the medication, I didn't feel one bit interested in sex. And I didn't feel any connection to Matt at this time. I felt like an empty shell. Sex seemed just too much to add to the mix.

I tried my best in this area to please him, to give him the love that usually came so easily to me, but it wasn't easy. I think it showed too. I could see the strain on Matt's face. I had gained so much weight from all the medication I didn't feel good about how my body looked. My cheeks were puffy, my hair was a dull color with no shine, my tummy was all distorted, which I am sure is the way many new moms feel, but I couldn't help but feel bad and unattractive.

I was getting to bed one night and Matt said, "*Hey Maggie, do you think your body will get back to the way it was?*" Immediately he knew that came out really wrong and tried to follow up with all kinds of nice statements. I heard it though, loud and clear. My mind became instantly dark, sad, and I just wanted to die right there. I was this ugly looking, overweight, mentally sick mother. How was I ever going to be sexy again?

In the mornings I would try my best to put on some make up and start making an effort with my coarse, dull hair. My sister Amy even came over and colored it for me because she knew I couldn't make it to a beauty salon chair. As she combed my hair I couldn't help but sit hopelessly still while the tears trickled out the corners of my eyes. How would I ever be beautiful again? How would my hair come back? How could I get this weight off? I wanted Matt to see me as the strong beautiful woman I once was. Only time would tell I guess. For now I had to be patient. Maybe dad was right about this God thing. He kept telling me daily on the phone it was on God's time not mine.

Chapter 24

The Black Cloud

As the days became weeks and the weeks became months my brain slowly began to heal. I still couldn't concentrate on following conversations well, television was a blur, and reading was downright impossible. It was very hard to deal with all the medication I was taking and be able to keep it all straight.

The side effects from the Abilify continued to plague me. My legs would shake constantly. By that I mean they never stopped moving. I told my doctor about this but she said I had to stay on the Abilify to make my brain calm. I felt like it was killing me a slow death.

After Christmas is definitely when the depression set in. I could feel it creeping in like a low, black fog. Here I was trying to come out of this stupid psychosis and now I was being handed a new battle.

At least the paranoia was dying off. I could feel myself losing hope of getting better. My body felt so rung out from having a baby, losing my identity, having major paranoia, and now I just felt sad.

I still had no connection to my baby. I wanted to love her, but I just didn't care about her. How could a mother not care about her little girl? How was this possible?

I was aware that I felt no connection to my baby and asked myself these questions every day. Of course when I was bombarded with these dark thoughts, my depression just got worse by the minute.

I called my mother one day in one of my dark moments trying so desperately to block out the bad thoughts racing through my brain. I sat on the kitchen floor dripping in sweat as I dialed my mom's number praying she would answer.

"*Hello*," my mom said in her sweet voice.

"*Mom,*" I said weakly. "*I am not having a good day. It is worse than usual. I am having such awful thoughts about myself, about Allison, Matt....I feel like I can't do this.*" I knew my mom could hear the desperation in my voice.

"*Margaret, I want you to call your doctor right now and get over there. Tell her everything you feel no matter how bad it is. Get it out. Call Anne for some help with Allison. I am going to send you a wood statue of Mary that you can hold. It is from a lady at my church and you can use it when you get real bad like this. I will go up to the post office right now and overnight it to you. Do you want me to come down? I will. Do you hear me? Margaret, I am talking to you right now! Are you listening to me?"*

"YES! Sorry I just have a hard time figuring out what you are saying. Yes, I will call Anne. I am so tired," I said quietly.

I had to do something. A thought of calling my best friend Carrie came to mind.

"Carrie!" I said urgently as she answered the phone. *"I need something to hang onto. I am having a desperate moment. Give me something,"* I stammered as I clenched my jaw tightly.

"Mag," Carrie said calmly. *"You are going to be okay. I have the perfect thing for you to hold onto,"* she said.

"You do? What is it? I am not doing well, Carrie," I said.

"Okay, this is what you are going to do, Mag." Carrie said.

"Get out a pencil and write this Bible verse down. Maggie, are you there? Maggie?" she said sternly.

"Yes, I have a pencil," I whispered back.

"Okay, so the verse is Philippians 3:13."

"Carrie, seriously, what is it, word for word? I can't look that up. I don't know where my Bible is. I haven't read it in years. Nor do I care to. That doesn't help! What else do you have? I am at my brink," I said. *"Plus, you already gave me that darn verse before!!*

"Mag, you just have to trust me on this. I am going to e-mail you the full verse, but right now I am going to read it to you and then tell you what it means, alright! You need to hear this verse again and again". I had no choice but to listen.

So she read Philippians 3:13. *"Brothers, I do not consider myself yet to have taken hold of it. But one thing I do: forgetting what is behind and straining toward what is ahead."* I was instantly transfixed by these powerful words, and I wanted more. They made me feel clear- headed for one small moment in time. It was as if some wave of peace had just washed over me.

"Carrie, I need you tell me in your words what this means?"

Carrie responded, *"Well, I think it means you need to focus your energy toward winning the race. You are the race. Your race is getting your family back together again.".*

I now was remembering my mother had told me the same thing a while back.

"Carrie, do you really think I will win the race?" I sobbed.

"Yep, I know you will," she says. *"It is going to be soon too. Now, before I go, I am going to pray for you."*

And so Carrie just did that. She said this perfect prayer that just felt so good. I could feel God's hand on me. I wasn't able to let him in just yet, but I wanted to.

I grew up being surrounded by God. My family went to church on Sundays, I went to Christian school for all my grade school years, sang all the church songs, and was in all the religious plays. I recited Bible verses during all my growing up years, but they never meant anything to me.

I had taken all these connections to God for granted and let them in, but just as effortlessly, let all my knowledge about God slip right out the other side. I was crippled by my mind telling me that I could do everything on my own. I didn't need help from some body or some being I couldn't see.

Listening to Carrie pray and bring me the word of God was the first time I felt something stir inside of me. It was as though the earth shifted. I could never go back to what was, and I didn't want to. I only needed more of what Carrie had just given me.

A peaceful feeling came over me and I wanted to hold my baby girl. I felt love all around me. I ran into our tiny little nursery and scooped up my darling little baby girl. "*I love you, baby girl!*" I cried. My tears flowed as she smiled up at me. "*You are so beautiful, little peanut. I feel like you are a gift.*"

That moment I experienced my first connection to my baby and to a feeling deep inside me that I didn't know was even possible.

Just then I heard the doorbell ring. That's right Anne was coming to save me. I hurried to the door with Allie cuddled in the crook of my arm.

"Maggie, you're holding Allison!" Anne said excitedly.

"Well, of course I am," I said. *"Why wouldn't I be?"*

"I was worried when you called this morning," Anne said.

"Oh yeah. That. I forgot how down I was this morning. My friend Carrie gave me this amazing Bible verse and it's helping. Strange, I know, but hey, whatever works!"

"Mom says I need to call my doctor about my depressing thoughts. So I guess I should follow up with that and get in to the doctor today. Can you come with me up to Del Mar? "

"*Sure,*" Anne says. "*Let's get your diaper bag packed and head up there.*"

Chapter 25

The Haze is Lifting

It was so strange sitting in my psychiatrist's office having a somewhat clear head. For once she was actually on time. Usually I would sit there waiting for at least 30-45 minutes, but today she had time to squeeze me in and she was on time!

Sitting on her burgundy couch, I looked at the decor on her walls. There was that big buffalo picture again that I stared at every time I sat in her office and of course that massive clock to the right of me, ticking way too loudly for my liking. I wish I could throw that stupid clock out the window.

The doctor had her psychiatrist certificate framed in front of me. She had gone to school in North Dakota. What the heck was out there? Maybe that is why she had buffalos on her walls. Just then the door opened and in she walked.

"*Hi Maggie. You are looking better,*" she said. "*Tell me, what is the urgency of today's visit? Talk to me.*"

"*Well, I had really bad thoughts today, like worse than usual. They are so bad I felt like I needed to kill myself.*" There. It was finally said, out in the open.

"*Maggie, I am glad you told me. We can fix this. We can adjust your medication and I think you need even more help around the house. Let's have a cleaning lady come in to help with laundry, getting the house in order, and even some cooking. We can get through this. The best thing about this is you got it out. Now that we know how bad your thoughts are, we can move forward to getting better,*" the doctor said.

She went into more depth about her plan and said she wanted me back three more times that week. I followed through on her request, making the 50 mile round trip in my Jeep with Anne and Allison riding in the backseat. Our trips up to the beautiful sleepy beach town were full of good talks and peaceful music I would play on my radio as I drove. Miraculously, it was as if I had been freed of the bad thoughts by speaking them out loud to my doctor.

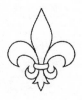

Chapter 26

Spring Training

I did what my psychiatrist instructed and found a housekeeper. She was a nanny who I met at Trolley Barn Park, just a few blocks from our house.

Ton was from Thailand, and she was employed by another family as a nanny. She was married to a counselor and did not know English well, but she had a wonderful personality. She loved having the extra money on top of her nanny job.

I could tell Ton missed her homeland because she would bring pictures from the village where she grew up. I could tell Ton was lonely too. She needed me as much as I needed her. Ton was good with baby Allison too. I would look forward to her coming every week to tidy up the house and get all the laundry done, which had always piled up.

Ton would even cook fresh, delicious Thai food for me and Matt. *"Maggie, I make you fresh rice and hot spicy soup. You eat! You need some good food to settle your nerves. You white people too nervous. This make you well,"* she would say in her broken English. As I was gulping down Ton's rice and soup, I heard Matt come in.

"Hi Mag," he called from the back bedroom. I knew he was scooping up Allison. He was all over her every chance he got. I was a bit jealous that he went to her first and not me. I guess I missed being number one. He used to always run to me and give me a kiss. Maybe this would all even out later on, but right now I felt as if I was coming in second place in a race, if I was being honest. I didn't like feeling this way and I knew my jealousy was dumb, so I tried to

set these feelings aside. At least I was actually having feelings for Matt again! I missed him. I missed what we had. This baby and my illness had created what felt like a huge abyss between us. How could we get back to being that perfect pair we had always been? I sighed out loud.

"You okay Maggie?" Ton asked.

"Yes, Thank you Ton. I just think too much," I said.

Ton gave me a puzzled response. I knew that look, the look that says 'what is wrong with you lady'? If only I could just be fine like all those other moms out there.

Matt walked into the kitchen. *"Hey Ton"*, Matt says. *"Maggie and I really appreciate all your hard work."* Matt paid her and walked her to the door, chatting all about Allie.

"So, Maggie, I have something I want to talk to you about," Matt said.

Oh no, this can't be good. What is he going to drop on me right now because I really don't think I can do whatever he asks? I felt so tired and out of it.

"I was talking with John Lowen today about maybe going out to Arizona for spring training. He said we could stay at his home during the weekend while we hit the games. I think it will be good for us to go on a little get-away. I already looked on Southwest Airlines and they are having great deals, plus Allie flies free."

Wow, I wasn't expecting this one. It was hard enough traveling ten hours all the way to Tahoe for a ski trip during Christmas. And now, getting on a flipping airplane. Well that just made my skin crawl.

In my head, I realized how awful this sounded so I responded with *"Why Matt, that sounds like a great idea."*

But I could feel the sweat start to bead up on my forehead just thinking about flying with a baby. Yes, the paranoia was gone at last, but I was still sick, hazy, emotional, and the fog of depression still hung heavily over me.

At the same time, I wanted to please Matt. I wanted him to be happy. So somehow I managed to put my own fears aside for him. I wanted my husband back so I was willing to dig down to the depths of my being and get ready for this trip.

As our plane sped down the runway in San Diego I gripped the armrests with all my strength while Matt held the bottle in Allie's mouth to help her ears adjust painlessly to the rapid change in altitude. He was so good with her. He made everything look so easy. Would I ever be a mom who could do what he was doing? Would I ever be able to make good decisions for Allie as he did?

My heart was racing as we became airborne. I guess we weren't going to crash but it sure felt like it.

I was stressed out for the entire flight. I was hoping Allie wouldn't cry, or make a sound. The flight attendants were at least helpful. They would come by and talk about how beautiful she was and ask me if I needed anything. But what I wanted they couldn't provide: to be in the safely of my home. Instead I was battling a massive panic attack, 30,000 feet in the air with no medication to calm me. I just had to muscle through it out and that was awful. By the time our short flight landed, I felt as I had lost three pounds in sweat.

Matt's friend John picked us up at the airport in Arizona. I think I called him in the first month after having Allison. It hit me right when I saw him. He knew how sick I was. He was a top ER doctor at some hospital here in Phoenix. I don't know what I had said to him in my deranged state in that phone call, but whatever it was he was very kind to me as he loaded all our stuff in his truck.

220

The Lowens' house was beautiful. It was a large two-story home with a nice pool in the backyard. He was living with his brother Jason at the time, who was in the business of flipping houses. Jason was Matt's roommate in college and John and Matt had attended high school so they were all very close.

John had a new girlfriend, Kerry, who was coming over in a little bit. I hoped I could act somewhat normal during dinner. We were planning to go out to dinner in a posh area of Arizona in the town of Scottsdale.

Later that night Kerry came to the house. She was delighted by Allison of course and was very nice to me as well. I instantly liked her. She was real to the core. Kerry was one of those people you feel you have known forever. She made everything seem easy and was smart as all get out. She was also an ER doc at the same hospital where John was finishing his residency.

Dinner was great but at the same time stressful. We ate at some yummy Mexican place with white lights above us on a beautiful patio. Scottsdale was full lights everywhere you looked. It was a tough balancing act that night trying to keep Allison happy, eat food when I could, and focus on a conversation with two doctors. Somehow I managed and made it to bed while I could hear Matt downstairs talking with John about tomorrow's games. I guess we were headed to see the Padres at 1pm game, in the heat of the day... great! This is not going to be good, I thought, and with that worry in mind, I passed out.

The next day we drove off to the stadium with a young baby, a full diaper bag, an anxious wife, and Matt and John talking in the front seat. As I had feared, we were right in the sun with the Mercury reading 95 degrees. I couldn't even manage 10 minutes in our seats, nor could Allison. She hated the sunscreen I tried to swab on her and started shrieking. I told Matt I had to go. Thank heavens he and John came up with a good plan. They found some seats away from the main crowd and in the shade.

The rest of the game I just checked out. I could have cared less about watching the Padres. By the time we got back to the house I was exhausted from the stress of the day. That night Kerry came over again and she and John cooked us dinner. They complemented each other so well and were cute together. They wore matching aprons that said "his" and "hers." I could definitely see them getting married.

I only wish I was more myself that night. I wanted Kerry to know the real me, not this over-anxious, rung-out mother who stood before her. I wonder what she thought of me? I really wanted her to like me. The next day was a double-header. I knew I couldn't make it. There is no way I was going to sit there again in that heat, with a baby and half a brain. Thankfully Matt agreed. He and John decided they would go and then leave a little early. That was great by me. I was freaking done!

The next day the boys went off to the game and I sat in the living room watching some crap on TV that I couldn't really follow anyway. Jason came in as I zoned out on some meaningless show. I was asking him all kinds of questions about his life and what he did.

Jason was not too into Allie. I could tell he was the bachelor type, into cute twenty-something girls, looking to have a good time, and not get into any serious relationships. He said he didn't want to end up married, bored with his wife, and stuck with kids. To top it off he said "*Hey, when you have kids, your wife goes downhill.*"

Great, is this what was happening to me? Was I becoming a drab, fat, out of shape, yucky wife in sweat pants? I looked down at myself and, yes, I was wearing a matching sweat suit. To my horror, I realized I was that person he had just described. How awful.

Despite Jason's saying this to a new mother, I know he didn't mean for me to take it personally or that he was trying to hurt my feelings. Nevertheless, what he said made me think hard. I wanted to get my old body back. I wanted to be out in the world again. I wanted my fun personality back, and to wear red lipstick again for Matt.

That night I gave Matt the best sex we had since we had Allison. It was the first time I wanted to be sexy again for my husband. I began to understand how difficult this process might be for any new mom. To try to balance a new baby in the household, to get your relationship back with your husband, and to figure out how you fit in this equation. It isn't easy even if you don't have Bipolar I.

On our flight home I started to feel a little bit more positive. Over the course of the following weeks, I was slowly weaned off the

Abilify, which was a huge feat in itself. Maybe there was a glimmer

of hope for me, for Matt, for our baby girl Allie.

Chapter 27

Prayer

During the weeks ahead, Anne and I got into a good rhythm dividing the mommy duties of taking care of Allie, and Ton and I divided household chores. Anne was a godsend, and my doctor had been right about getting more help. Ton's help with the laundry and prepping meals alleviated a lot of my stress, allowing me to concentrate on my main job of getting well. I was trying very hard to get better with ever-clearer focus on the end goal of being in charge and having my family to myself. As when I raced competitively, keeping my eye on the prize was an effective motivator that worked for me.

I now wanted to be with Allie on my own like other mothers. Anne had been helping me for seven months now and she had taught me everything about how to take care of a newborn. She had Allie and Me on a strict schedule everyday. I think that was key too. When Allie would go down for her naps, I would nap too. I usually wanted to get tons of stuff done while Allie slept, but Anne insisted that this was my chance to use the rest to keep getting well. And she was right too because I began to heal a little bit everyday.

Maybe my dad and Carrie were right about God having a hand in this. I decided to start praying. To say my prayers every night as I did when I was a little girl might just help. I know Matt's mom Donna had her entire church praying for me. She was a true prayer warrior. I still wondered though, if God was truly a kind and just God, why had he made me go through this living hell? What had I done to possibly deserve this illness that gave me such an awful start to being a mother?

This question would pop into my mind often, especially when I observed other mothers out with their babies, looking happy and at ease. When I was out with Allison running errands at a store, I would notice them having such an easy time, with their strollers, and perhaps a friend or mom helping out, all laughing while they did their shopping.

On the other hand, it was a massive struggle for me to make it to any store. I was slow due to the medication still being pumped through my system and would wonder up and down the aisles looking at outfits for Allie and tons of baby stuff that didn't interest me. I so badly wanted to be one of the at-ease mothers who seemed to enjoy these gadgets and cute little clothes. Grocery shopping was even worse. I wanted relief from this hell that my mind was trapped in.

The worst was going anywhere with Allie in the car. Just getting Allie into her car seat wore me out. Every time I buckled her in, it would take me many frustrating minutes because I couldn't remember how to do it. Anne wouldn't help me because she wanted me to learn on my own. She stood by, but did less and less, trying to boost me into independence. I wanted it badly myself, but struggled at the same time.

I started my prayers early in the morning. I could hear Matt getting ready for work and carrying Allie, having an entire conversation with her. I wanted to be a part of their fun world. I wanted to be talked to too. I yelled, *"Matt can you come in her for a minute?"*

"Sure Mag," he called back. Just then he came in holding our cute little baby. I was indeed starting to fall in love with this little one.

"Matt, can you pray for me?"

"*Maggie,*" he said. "*I have been praying for you every day and night. In fact I will pray for you this very moment.*"

As he prayed for me out loud with Allie cuddled in his arms I could feel a tremendous amount of peace. I also could feel hot tears rolling down my cheeks. God was here with my little family. I could feel it. I didn't have the close relationship with Him that Matt did, but I would. Something was starting to stir down in that stubborn heart of mine.

After Matt left for work, I went over and dressed Allie for the day and took her over to the rocking chair. "*God,*" I said out loud. "*I pray for myself to heal. I want to be a great mother. I want my old life back. I want to be on my own again. Please heal my brain so I can achieve this goal. Amen.*"

I opened my eyes and Allie was looking at me with all smiles. I couldn't help but giggle and laugh at the cute chubby little face. She cooed at me back. I just sat and rocked with her until

Anne came and the day began.

Chapter 28

Carrie's Checkup

The next week Carrie came down for a visit. It was so nice to see her and be able to be more clear-headed than the previous times she had been around. Half her visits in the past year had been a blur when I could hardly figure out how to communicate with her.

I cleaned my tiny house and eagerly awaited Carrie's arrival. Now that Allie had one of our two bedrooms, our oversized red velvet couch had become our guest room. As I made some sweet tea I could hear Jackson barking in the front yard. That must be

Carrie. I peeked through the curtain and sure enough there she was in her white pickup trying to calm down our excited Labrador.

"*Carrie,*" I said called from our front door.

"*Hey Mags*", she replied. "*Glad to see that smile on your face.*"

Everyone kept talking about my smile. I guess it had been absent so long it was good for everyone to see it back again.

"*Where is that baby of yours?*" she said. "*Allie has probably gotten quite big since I was last down. Those kids grow like weeds, don't they?*"

"*Yes, Carrie,*" I said. "*Something like plants all right. She is napping at the moment. She still takes two naps a day.*"

"*It's my break time for myself,*" I tell her. "*Go ahead and take a peek!*"

She does and I can tell she just loves Allie. We are going to have a lot of fun with this kiddo when she gets older. With Carrie and me being huge sports fans, Allie better like sports too. We head

for my deck behind the house and have some sweet tea as Jackson

lies at my feet.

"*So what have you been up to, Mag, besides being here with*

baby?" Carrie asks.

"*Well, a lot,*" I respond. I fill her in quickly with the day-to-

day mommy baby lifestyle I had become apart of. She listens with

infinite support and patience. I know my life must seem boring

compared to Carrie's. She is a professor at Azusa Pacific University

and the head softball coach there as well.

I tell Carrie about my interest in all this religious stuff that

keeps running through my head. With that she is listening even

more intently.

"*So Mag, maybe while I am here this weekend we should try*

church? I know this church called The Rock which is right here by your home and Miles McPherson is the head Pastor. He was a San Diego Charger back in his day." Well, that sounded not so bad.

"I think that is the church my friend Cherlynn attends," I said. *"I will see if she will come with us."*

Little did I know I was on the road to the first peace I would ever feel in my life.

The rest of the day we played with Allie, took her on her daily walk to the cute little Trolley Barn Park that I loved, and even stopped for a yummy coffee drink at a cafe that was only a block from my house.

Matt was happy Carrie was down for the weekend too. Out of all the friends I had ever introduced Matt to, nobody came close to Carrie. She knew what was happening on just about any topic, which Matt loved, especially sports, which impressed Matt the most. Plus, on top of that, she was an incredible cook. That night she cooked us her famous tacos, which we devoured with gusto and

I was thankful for the much-needed break in the kitchen. Gone were the days where we would just go out to dinner if we were tired. I had to cook every night.

By the time Sunday rolled around, I was really looking forward to my first time in a church in years. Matt and I had attended a Presbyterian church for a number of years after we were married when we lived at the beach but I never really felt connected and only went because I thought we should, not because I felt the need. I was able to throw together a nice skirt and top and even make my hair look nice. Matt stayed home with Allison so I could concentrate on the outing. Cherlynn showed up right on time and off we went.

Part Three: Shambling Toward the Finish Line

Chapter 29

I Believe

As we drove to the church I oddly felt an excitement in me and not the sad distant shell I had been living in. There were hundreds of cars in the parking lot. This was the craziest thing I had ever seen. All these people heading to church obviously liked what they were hearing or getting from it. Maybe there was hope for me here or maybe I was chasing some unforeseen channel.

People welcomed us as we walked in and took our seats. I tried to study the program they handed me but I could not concentrate on the words. I could hardly wait until the day I was able to read again. It was a part of this illness. When my brain goes

into Mania or Depression, reading becomes almost impossible.

Carrie and Cherlynn sat on either side of me, which felt good. It

was like there was so much love in the room I felt utterly

overwhelmed with comfort deep inside me.

There was a band up on the stage and they started up their

music as the congregation stood. The music was incredible. I didn't

know the words but wanted to sing right along with everyone else.

Carrie and Cherlynn knew the songs well and were belting them

out with joy and pride. I looked up on the screen and sang as best I

could.

I felt again something stir deep in my soul. A soul I thought

didn't exist. A soul that was lost and one I thought that could never

be found. The more we sang these praise songs to God the more I

could feel the barriers begin to break.

As Miles McPherson begun to preach I began to listen. He talked of getting to know God in a personal way, taking him as your rock, accepting him as your Christ and Savior. Christ and Savior.

What was all this? I locked onto the entire sermon. Before, in church my brain would just wonder and I would go through the motions. Now I wanted to take action and I wanted it today. One verse I copied down was James 1:2-6: *"Consider it pure joy, my brothers, whenever you face trials of many kinds because you know that the testing of your faith develops perseverance. Perseverance must finish its work so that you may be mature and complete, not lacking anything. If any of you lacks wisdom, he should ask God, who gives generously to all without finding fault, and it will be given to him. But when he asks, he must believe and not doubt, because he who doubts is like a wave of the sea, blown and tossed by the wind."*

There was that same verse Carrie had had me write down months earlier. This was crazy! And the freaking trials. I felt like my trials were beyond trials.

I had had enough of this fighting Bipolar on my own. I was done. I needed somebody else to guide me through this battle. Right then and there I knew I needed God to be in charge. I no longer wanted to doubt Him and be tossed with the wind and seas. I wanted in. I wanted Christ at my center. I didn't know how this would happen but I knew I was hungry and thirsty for God for the first time in my life.

Pastor McPherson started to wrap up his sermon and ask if there was anybody in the Church who wanted to accept Christ in their life. I wanted to stand and shout ME! As he went on about having Christ as your Lord and Savior I started to tremble and tears were gushing down my face. He asked those who wanted God to stand.

I whispered in Carrie's ear, *"I don't want to stand, but I want God in my heart!"*

"Maggie, you don't have to stand," Carrie said. *"God knows."*

I sat there with my eyes closed listening to the Pastor and accepting Christ at last to take my life into His own hands. It had taken me 31 years to get there but at last I had come to the party.

I felt so much relief as Jesus came over me. The control that I had held onto on my own all these years was utterly exhausting and now I had handed the baton over to Him and I was glad. I knew that day I was no longer alone fighting Bipolar. I no longer had to worry about death, destruction, depression, mania, my baby Allison, and Matt. Christ was in charge and He alone would see to it that we were taken care of.

I couldn't wait to get home to tell Matt. Carrie and Cherlynn gave me hugs and they too had tears in their eyes. They knew what this was like. They had been through their own journeys that I had never cared to ask them about and now I wanted to know.

Why hadn't I listened all these years? Now it made sense why Cherlynn was such a kind and caring person no matter what. She had God in her heart.

As for Carrie, I had known her all my life and remembered she had become a Christian in her late college years but I thought she had lost her mind. Now I understood why she was a counselor at all those Christian camps during the summers. She was sharing God with others. She was sharing her joy and knowledge with people like me that just were not getting it.

Chapter 30

Change

After the massive barrier I had broken, my life began to change in every way imaginable. It was like God was saying, "*fly Maggie!*" He was telling me to concentrate on what was important. He was telling me to give Him the worries and enjoy this bundle of love Allison.

Matt was so excited about this new change in me. I no longer worried Matt might die at work, that we would run out of money, and that I would be a bad mom. I still had a long way to go in healing my brain but now there was a newfound hope. I had hope that I had never had before. A close bond was forming with my baby girl Allison.

Things were doing so well that it was time for Anne to leave us of all things. I would miss her dearly but she was no longer needed. Plus she was breaking my mother's and Matt's parents' bank accounts. She had done her part in making sure our little one was safe while I got well. Here we all were coming out of the trenches once again as a whole family. So many awful things could have happened.

They say it takes a village. This village was a massive force to fight a Bipolar psychosis postpartum episode. We all fought this together with everything we had and with God at the helm we persevered.

Chapter 31

Beach Celebration

My mother was so happy the way things were progressing; she came up with the idea of a week's celebration together at the beach. We stayed in the Back Bay Area of Mission Beach in a condo. Matt's family and mine all stayed together and celebrated making it through this awful storm.

As I sat on the beach with Allie taking in the sun I could feel God's warmth filling me up through my insides. He was indeed in charge now. I no longer had the crazy-making stress I had endured my entire life.

Of course I would always have Bipolar disorder, but now I had somebody bigger than myself to lean on. When the suicidal thoughts would creep in, I now could look to God with prayers. I could also turn to my Christian friends, my mom, my mother-in-law Donna, my best friend Carrie, and most of all my husband who had been patiently waiting all these years for me to become a Christian.

Matt had been through so much this year. A year of hell in the form of a shell of a wife who was either distraught, in depends diapers, forgot how to shower, or eat. It didn't matter though; he had waited for me. He had prayed for me and loved me no matter how dark things had been.

I looked down at baby Allison munching on sand. She was wearing a bright orange bikini that my sister had put her in with a big white floppy baby that the Lowens had given me. I laughed out loud and yelled at Matt to look at Allie. He came running out of the bay and scooped her up and washed her off, laughing all the way.

My mom and dad and Jim laughed too. This was starting to feel as it should. We were all a family again in a healthy way. Just then Donna emerged from her swim and was also delighted by all of us laughing together. The week continued with all of us eating, playing games, and swimming daily. I felt truly blessed to have this family never give up on me.

Chapter 32

A New Identity

The peaceful, sunny days seemed to fly by fast. Matt was

with me the entire time since he was out for the summer because he

was a teacher.

As fall rolled around it was starting to feel a little rough for

me again. I no longer had the mania, postpartum stuff, but now

was dealing with what a normal mother might face. It was this

awful feeling of where I belonged again. I was so alone. I knew

there were other new moms out in the world like me but I didn't know how to reach them. At the park I went to it was full of nannies so I didn't even know where to begin there.

I was overjoyed when Matt came home with a paper telling me about mommy groups I could go to. It made me very nervous but yet excited. I needed outside contact to get through this. I needed some new friends. I wanted to know how others were doing and wanted to learn more about being a mom.

I was getting better about taking care of Allie's needs now. I could now change her diaper, feed her, tend to all her needs, and nap her throughout the day.

I tried my best to put on an outfit that was kind of cute, fixed my hair, and makeup. I got everything I thought I might need for our first big outing on our own to the mommy meet-up playdate.

It felt as though I was going to the biggest interview of my life. My brain felt muddled and on overload. How was I going to be able to meet people and feel like I had something in common? I had just spent the past seven months of my life in what felt like a coma with no connection to people or my baby for heavens sake. I put on some designer jeans that were called 7's. My mother had bought them for me telling me they were the hot new item. With my fashion background it was so weird to not know what was "in". Well at least I would hit this mom event with style.

My hands were shaking as I packed Allie's diaper bag. I was insanely nervous about this. Going to a park full of moms and babies just downright terrified me. I knew I had to do this though. Matt was so right about taking this needed step. It was time to emerge from the safety of my house and graduate from watching depressing lifetime movies all day.

I arrived at the park right on time and saw other moms already there with their cute blankets and diaper bags making everything look so easy. I put Allie in her cute little pink stroller and slowly headed to the group. Some moms were on their blankets talking while their children played on the play structure while others ran after theirs. I felt so completely out of place. Just then a mom looked up at me and smiled.

"Hi, I am Ali," she said kindly. *"Nice to meet you,"* I managed to say. *"Great name you have there, that is my daughter's name."*.

I set my stuff down next to Ali and was able to wiped the sweat off my brow. Much to my relief I was starting to ease up a bit just by meeting Ali. She was so friendly and was talking to some other moms who also introduced themselves to me. It was nice to hear their complaints about how difficult it was for them at home. It made me realize that I wasn't the only one out there with difficulties.

There were others trying to figure out this tough road out there. Maybe they didn't start out with my same problems but theirs were very tough too, just in different ways. One had a near death experience during childbirth, another had bad health problems right after she got home with her new baby, and yet another was from the Midwest and moved out here knowing nobody.

The girl from the Midwest was only 24 years old. Wow, I thought, so brave to be so far from her home, married to a military guy she met while she was in the Navy and chasing her 15 month old around the slides. She was very quiet but right from the start I could tell we had a lot in common. We shared the same political views, liked a lot of the same books, and she made me feel normal most of all.

Her name was Kelly. Her daughter, Alexa, was hilarious to watch. She had a big fluff of blond hair and had so much energy. She was crawling on everything she laid eyes on. Allie liked following Alexa, which was pretty cute in itself. The two hours flew by with us sitting on the blankets talking about our lives and feeding our children.

That evening I was actually waiting by the door with a smile when Matt walked in.

"Maggie, do I see a smile?" he asked. *"I see a light in your eyes, I haven't seen in a long time. Tell me. What's up?"*

"Well Matt, I did what you said," I said. *"I attended to my first mom meet up outing."*

I told him all about the different nice moms that I met, and the other babies and small children that were there. I could tell he was pleased that I was finally engaging with others. He was starting to see his wife return to him.

From that first meeting on, I began to keep a calendar of the events I wanted to attend. We had all kinds of different meeting places. Going to Sea World or the San Diego Zoo with a bunch of strollers and moms became a highlight of my week. It was a reason to put fun outfits and makeup on. Most of all I enjoyed being able to talk to other moms.

The mommy groups were such an outlet for me. I began to emerge from my depression and come to life each time I attended. The moms there had no idea how much they were my therapy, my saving grace.

Kelly and I began to meet each other for play dates outside of the mommy groups. I only lived 15 minutes from her home in Point Loma. Her house was practically across the street from the little business I used to run called Maggie's Skin Care. What a lifetime ago that was. A life when I was making money on a daily basis, would go out to lunch all the time with friends, and meet Matt for a drink after work.

That life seemed like it had happened to a different person. It was so strange how much my complete identity could change in a year. I went from social working girl to stay-at-home deranged

Mom. At least I could start to see hope now in this new occupation of mine. It was only months earlier that I could hardly get out of bed to greet the day.

The play dates with Kelly were so comfortable. She didn't mind that I had this illness Bipolar that I was greatly affected by. She just accepted for who I was. Our little ones would play with toys or we would put them in their strollers and head to the cute little marketplace that was within walking distance of her house. We would often go to Panera Bread and sit and have a bowl of broccoli cheddar soup and talk about what we wanted to do with our girls' rooms, or how we might decorate our living rooms.

I met another girl I really clicked with in the group as well. Her name was Jamie. She also got along well with Kelly. Jamie was sweet to the core and never had a bad thing to say about anybody. She was a no-drama girl, which meshed well with me. The three of us would often hang out together at the meet-ups and also would do fun lunches out with our kiddos in tow outside the group.

There was something about Jamie that I needed to know more about. As I hung out with her more and more over the next few months I was intrigued about where she would focus her energy and thoughts. She would toss in the conversation from time to time about how much her church had helped her and how she had Jesus in her heart. I found this interesting since Carrie had kept me hanging on these Bible verses for help over the past year. I had accepted Jesus in my life but now I wasn't following up. I knew this was my next step. I knew it was time to start going to church.

One my way to Kelly's I passed by a large truck that had JESUS IS LORD painted on the side in huge letters. It was so strange; sayings like these kept jumping out at me.

Jesus wouldn't leave my mind. Jesus is Lord. This is why I needed to go to church. I needed to know what all this meant.

I now believed in God, but didn't know why or how He would interact in my daily life. I needed more information. I needed instruction on this journey I was headed on. Why was I thinking about this? Stuff like this had never had never bothered me before. Why now, was the continuing question in my mind?

The following week I talked Matt into going to Jamie's church in Claremont. I was taken aback by the kindness of the congregation. Everyone there was friendly and helpful. I knew now this would be the next step in my journey to getting to know Christ better. Claremont Covenant, the Pastor, Greg West, Matt, and Allie in my arms would help me continue to stay on this path all the way to getting baptized years later.

Chapter 33

The Bend at the Blackfoot

I would eventually finish and publish my first book called

Runaway Mind in 2009. I stood up in front of my church and

delivered my first speech on Bipolar and my faith to 200 people in

this church. My church congregation bought my book and

supported me every step along the way through my ups and downs.

I had a book event in my hometown of Sonora and signed and sold

books for three hours straight at the Mountain Bookshop.

The title of my first speech was *"Walk By Faith not By*

Sight." This Bible verse 2 Corinthians 5:7 was my brother's very

first memory verse in school. It was what my father told me in the depths of my despair. When my pastor had me speak before the church congregation he spoke of this verse, which my entire talk was about. God had set up this never-ending theme for my life. I needed to keep walking by my faith in Christ not by what I saw around me!

I continued to speak all over San Diego, helping others with Bipolar, and received awards for my mental health advocacy work. I was interviewed on radio programs, and even had my own radio show with Tanya Brown, Nicole Brown Simpson's sister, about mental illness. Newspaper articles were written about my work. I received letters from all over the world on how I helped a daughter, son, mother, father, wife, husband, or friend.

My Bipolar would not become my life though. My life had been set free. My main job now to be a wife and mother, to enjoy and raise my daughter, Allison, and be a happy wife once again.

I took Allie everywhere with me. We would set out on my surfboard together or ride our bikes. We traveled to Hawaii with Matt's parents. We went to my parents' ranch and rode the tractor with Mom and walked the ranch with Dad. Allie learned to ride a horse. Matt bought us a beautiful home in Poway with an acre and a swimming pool Allie would have big parties with all her friends. Matt planted a backyard vineyard and remodeled our house with his cousin, big John IV.

I even began working again, doing massage, after Allie started school. One client in particular, a gracious mature lady, named Mrs. Helen Anne Bunn helped me make my faith even stronger and gave me confidence to be the mom I wanted to become. She eventually helped me set up my own business again, doing massages and facials out of my home.

We found a loving community at a new church called Green Valley right by our home. We never wanted to miss a Sunday service.

Matt and I made new friends who supported us in every way, friends we could rely on if I was having a bad day to swoop in and drop off dinner or help with laundry. We traveled to Montana with the Lowens and stayed on the famous Blackfoot River with their new baby girl, Eva. Matt would fly-fish with John every day while I finished this book.

Right now, as I sit on the porch of the Kerry family's log cabin I can spot Matt and John in the distance, flipping their poles back and forth across the big bend of the Blackfoot, trying to catch that perfect trout. I feel truly at peace out in the middle of nowhere on this 70-acre paradise.

As I look up from this real dream I can't help but think of how so many people gave up time in their lives for Allie, Matt, and me. I think most of all of how Jesus sacrificed his life to give me eternal life.

I may have some very hard days ahead still, but now I have Jesus in my heart. When you get down to it, that is all the truly matters.

When I die I will go to heaven and be with Jesus forever. A place with no Bipolar sounds like heaven to me.

I can hear something to the side of me and a doe emerges from the bushes and stops and stares at me. I feel at peace just staring back. She then bounds back into the brush as little Eva and Allie come running out on to porch. Kerry comes out after them.

"*Well Maggie, lets go hit the river,*" Kerry says.

We join the boys at the bend of The Blackfoot River and ruin any chance of their hopes of catching the big one.

A Mother-in-Law Painfully Remembers

By Donna Reese

I got the phone call from our son when they were at the hospital and Maggie was in labor.

How exciting! Our second granddaughter was exercising her way into this world and ours. First babies weren't supposed to come three weeks early, and my thoughts were elsewhere that Wednesday morning, October 3rd 2006. My head spun with figuring out a way to travel over 400 miles and get there in time for her delivery. I went into a flurry of disorganized packing, got a good weather report, headed to our small local airport in central California, and flew myself to San Diego. The sun was setting as I drove the rental car to the hospital with baby girl thoughts happily tumbling around in my mind.

Even though I missed the delivery by a few hours, the new little family were bonded and happy and doing just great. Maggie was such a loving and devoted little mama and nursing Allie easily and naturally. Allison had big bright blue eyes and was tiny, but perfect. Proud new dad, Matt, adapted immediately with pride and pleasure to his new role as Daddy. My Grammy heart sang praises to our Heavenly Father for a safe delivery, a healthy baby and joyous new family.

Everyone on the maternity ward knew and loved Maggie in the few short days she was there. Her magnetic personality drew people to her. The day nurse became a new best friend. People seemed to go out of their way to care for Allison and Maggie--the new darlings of the ward.

Everything seemed to be going well, but then the questions started to creep in: Is this the normal euphoria of a mom experiencing the joy of a new babe in arms? Or, is this -- do I dare even think it in my mind -- the manic symptoms of a new bipolar mother? No! No!! I can't even allow that thought to pass through, or speak it to another. As I cuddled our beautiful granddaughter, I brushed all those terrible questions aside.

My husband, Papa Jim, arrived that evening and shared the joyous event and celebrated the family's blessings. His foreboding thoughts matched mine, although we didn't speak it until the following day. Wound up in a manic whirlwind, Maggie talked fast and jumped from one topic to the next without a breath. Matt was beginning to come to terms with the same internal thoughts. Discharged from the hospital, Maggie was breaking away from reality--slipping out of sight. She was unable to bond with Allison. She was aware that she needed to get back on her bipolar medications (discontinued during pregnancy), but the psychiatrist didn't answer our calls, return calls, or have any psychiatrist covering patients. We were helpless to get a prescription. Manic Maggie was falling over the Reality Edge and we all could see it escalating quickly, yet were helpless to stop the downward spiral.

So we went to the Emergency Room with hopes of obtaining the appropriate medications. Two choices were offered: 1. Admit Maggie to the psychiatric ward or 2. See her psychiatrist. The psychiatrist still was not responding, so there was o real help there.

Maggie was lying down in the back of the car with her eyes closed and when she spoke, her words tumbled out incoherently. I prayed, "HELP us Lord. We don't want this new mother locked up and separated from her baby." We had little resources to deal with the surmounting odds.

Papa Jim's training as a physician and surgeon, calls for decisive action when no immediate medical intervention is available. Jim contacted an experienced psychiatrist practicing in another state, and he was a huge help in providing a free phone consultation and giving his professional opinion of medications he would recommend for Maggie. With a leap of faith and a prayer, Dr. Jim called in the prescriptions for Maggie, with the blessing of Matt, and Joe and Leslie. Holding our breath, we waited and prayed.

Running a Home-Based Psychiatric Ward and Nursery is not for the faint of heart. Plunging in with helping hands and hearts, nothing could have prepared us for this challenging non stop work week. It was a blur of prepping, feeding, diapering, laundry, cleaning, cooking, coaching, counseling, praying, worrying, encouraging, etc.

Allison was an easy baby and took far less time to tend to than her sick mother. We hoped Allison was oblivious to the anxiety, paranoia, and worries of death her mom experienced.

Beautiful Maggie's personal grooming skills disappeared. It became a huge challenge for her to brush her teeth, change clothing, or shower. Her fear of drowning in the bath made her pretend she had washed, rather than face those very oppressive fears of death. How long must she suffer? When would the meds make a visible difference?

We became micro managers of her existence, trying to love her back into the real world. Maggie had no ability to read, concentrate, or focus on even the simplest tasks.

This vibrant woman, who could work circles around all her friends, was incapable of anything productive. How I missed her creative energy and sparkling personality. They were gone. She was more like a Zombie than a young new mother.

We placed Allie in Maggie's arms and she held her dutifully, yet was completely unresponsive to her darling daughter. A five pound sack of flour would have received equal attention--none.

There was no bonding or recognition that this infant was her very own.

Sometimes her vacant eyes stared; then, suddenly, they would fervently dart about as her psychotic brain dreamt of horrible happenings. She talked about Matt being dead and people spying on us. As much as we reassured or shared scripture or prayed with her, the Evil Thoughts were her reality. Maggie spoke the truth about knowing these things were not real, yet, as hard as she fought to believe that, the images were bigger than she could dismiss.

Matt came home from his high school teaching job worn out and faced the Psych Ward Wife. He was tender, loving, and patient with her, and took over the night feedings for his "Baby Blue Eyes." He did not express his fears or reveal his emotions, but as his mother, I ached for him, the pain visible on his drawn face. Laughter was absent in this Hospital House. Joy of a newborn baby was smashed down by the heaviness of a new mother and wife gone mad.

How long would it take for Maggie to "come back."? Would she regain her ability to function as a normal, safe person? How long could the Psych Ward be carried out in a home setting? Who do you call when Humpty Dumpty is broken and all the King's Men are gone? I would crawl into bed exhausted, wondering when was the last time I had a chance to brush my hair and teeth--two days? Sleep was difficult and restless, but I would take whatever snippets I could get.

Mornings would bring renewed hope. We were on a mission to find a doula to help in this healing process. The normal function of a doula is to help during labor and delivery in a non-medical capacity. Some doulas stay with their clients for a few weeks to help them get the baby established on a schedule. We needed a Miracle Doula who would be willing to do that and much more.

The calls and interviews took place. It was easy to check "no" to all the applicants -- except one. Ann was calm and confident and understood Maggie's mental health status and that her role would be one of training Maggie to become a competent, safe, mother. She was an answer to our prayers, our Angel Doula. Ann began her work several weeks later, mentoring Mama Maggie for the next five months.

Today, life ebbs and flows like the San Diego beaches that Matt, Maggie, and Allie freely explore and play in. Allie is a smart, beautiful, active, athletic, fun, healthy fourth grade girl. Her mom and dad flex well with the ebb and flow of life. There are way more good days than down days. My beautiful daughter-in-law is involved, active, energetic, and creative. She has decorated and landscaped their home in marvelous ways. She and Matt are the glue that make a lovely, safe home for Allison. This family trio are active in church and social activities and enjoy exploring their world. They are a team. They know what life was like at the depths of hell, but their faith has sustained them through those tough times and holds them steady in the good times.

This faith journey is ongoing and we have all grown closer to God and one another through these deep emotional and difficult times. We celebrate life with the knowledge, "For we walk by faith, not by sight." (I Corinthians 5:7, KJV). We know "...With man this is impossible, but with God all things are possible." (Matthew 19:26). We can face today and tomorrow with great confidence because of Isaiah 41:10: "So do not fear, for I am with you; do not be dismayed, for I am your God. I will strengthen you and help you; I will uphold you with my righteous right hand."

Take Two

A Loyal Best Friend Through Thick and Thin but not

Again

By Maggie's best friend, Carrie Webber

God's plan for your life can be a mystery. Sometimes it's a great adventure and crazy mystery all in one. One you enjoy the entire time and can't wait to see what He will do next. I like those journeys, those mysteries that keep you on the edge of your seat. I love trusting God with my life and letting Him guide my day to day. And, then there's those "other" journey's. Those other mysteries of life that you wish would just end and be done. Where you don't understand what God is doing, or why He is doing it. Why is He allowing these crappy and awful things to happen to you and the people you love? Why? Seriously! What is the point?

The last time I sat down to write about Maggie and her journey through her first major Bipolar break I figured it would a one-and-done type of thing. I would write a few words of how it affected me, and then we would go about our lives like usual. Well, that's not how life works out most of the time. Allow me for a brief moment to be cliché in my scripture usage. But there is a reason things are "cliché," and it's usually because it's relevant and it happens all the time. In God's word he tells us:

"I have told you these things, so that in me you may have peace. In this world you will have trouble. But take heart. I have overcome the world." John 16:33"

What sticks out to me is that blunt and truthful statement that I WILL have trouble. I will have problems, sickness, stress, heartache, trouble, hard decisions, death and a multitude of other things make our lives miserable.

So every time I ask God "Why?" I need not look any further than this word. Our world is fallen and full of turmoil, so don't be surprised when something bad happens to you or the people you love. God says it will happen, but he gives us hope. Jesus Christ came, died, and rose from the dead. He conquered death itself in order that it has no power over us. No matter what heartache we face in this life we have the promise of victory in heaven. So you see, I didn't ask "why?" when Maggie got sick the first time. And I didn't ask "why?" when she got sick after having Allison. I simply asked God to help us through this trial. To give us doctors with wisdom who could help Maggie. And give us enough strength to take care of our selves and Maggie and Allison. To gently speak to Maggie and show her His awesome grace and agape love to her. To show her that the only way to get through this life is with Him by her side.

It's all I wanted for her at this point in her life. Life is hard enough even when you are healthy and happy, but throw in some bi-polar and life is a complete manic disaster. God wants us to have peace in the midst of every storm, just like the verse says above. So that's what I prayed. Every day, without fail I got on my knees and asked that God would show Maggie how to live this life with Him as her strength and guide.

So, does God really need me to pray to Him in order for Him to reveal himself to Maggie? Not really. He already knows what's going on and what needs to be done. But he created us to be in relationship with him and that means talking to him. He wants us to talk to him as you would to your mom or dad or best friend. He actually commands us to pray in order to be a part of what He's doing and experience Him in a way that is only done through prayer. Jesus, the Son of God, prayed constantly to his Heavenly Father. He was showing us what was important and how to impact people here on earth through the God of the universe. So, yeah, I was all about talking to God about Maggie. I wanted my friend back and I wanted her back fully. She needed to come back to us, and not for us, but for her little precious baby girl.

I love Maggie with all my heart. I would lay down my life for my friend. She is a remarkable person who was blessed with a personality that could handle Bipolar. Not everyone could do what she has done and come through it as well as she has. But you see, she grabbed onto the life ring that was thrown to her. But this time God was throwing and pulling her in to the shore. Her family and friends were standing on the firm ground cheering her on as they have always done. She allowed the waves of grace to wash over her and release her from having to shoulder this life on her own. She was drowned in God's love and hope for her life. And she now stands on the firm foundation of Jesus Christ. A foundation that's unshakeable and one you won't slip from. You can't make this stuff up. You just can't. We pray so that we can be apart of what God is doing. And this was a miracle in my book, a miracle that I was witness to and got to share with the rest of the world. So never underestimate the power of prayer. My Maggie is living proof that "with God, all things are possible." Matthew 19:26

Oh, one last thing though. Let's not do this again!

Afterword

I asked Matt for a quote for this book, *"What do you want me to say Mag? I had two diapers to change. It was like having twins. It was hell."*

When Allie was four years old, she came up with a joke that she said I could use at the NAMI Awards dinner. *"So, Mommy. I was thinking. I was the peanut, Dad is the walnut, and you are the cracked nut!"* The joke was a hit when I made my thank you speech for San Diego NAMI Advocate of the Year."

Bipolar has been hard on me, but it has been even harder on my family. When I've been out of it, they still are aware of what is going on, and suffering greatly because of it.

Allie and I have been talking about my illness since she learned to talk. I think it is important that children know what is going on. They are smarter then we all might think, right. She knows when I am having an off day and gives me space or says she is going to pray real hard for me. Even though I lost my mind once again after I gave birth, now I have this amazing daughter in my life.

Allie is now eight years old. How can time go so fast? I learn something from her everyday. She is an incredible gift God has blessed me with.

People often ask me if I would have done anything different? I think if I had the money I would have used a surrogate mother. There are just so many risks in having a baby with

Bipolar. There's such a crappy reality staring in the face of all women with Bipolar who want to be moms. Motherhood can be done, but my best advice is to set up your team of who will come to help you – early!

I have already started my third book on my life. I can't help it. There is always something happening and never a dull moment. I guess it is in me to write. I look over at Matt and he is sleeping soundly next to me. I need to get to bed. Life goes on.

RESOURCES

IF URGENT HELP IS NEEDED

If you are in crisis, facing an emergency, if you fear that you may harm yourself, your baby or others you need to immediately call your healthcare provider, dial 911, go to the nearest hospital emergency room or contact a qualified crisis line, such as the National Suicide Prevention

Suicide Prevention

National Hopeline Network

1-800-SUICIDE (1-800-784-2433)

http://www.hopeline.com

National Suicide Prevention Lifeline:

1-800-273-TALK (1-900-273-8255)

http://www.suicidepreventionlifeline.org

Edinburgh Postnatal Depression Scale 1 (EPDS)

Name: _____ Address: _____

Your Date of Birth: _____ _____

Baby's Date of Birth: _____ Phone: _____

As you are pregnant or have recently had a baby, we would like to know how you are feeling.

Please check the answer that comes closest to how you have felt IN THE PAST 7 DAYS, not just how you feel today.

Here is an example, already completed.

I have felt happy:

Yes, all the time

Yes, most of the time - This would mean: "I have felt happy most of the time" during the past week.

No, not very often - Please complete the other questions in the same way.

No, not at all

In the past 7 days:

1. I have been able to laugh and see the funny side of things *6. Things have been getting on top of me

As much as I always could Yes, most of the time I haven't been able

Not quite so much now to cope at all

Definitely not so much now Yes, sometimes I haven't been coping as well

Not at all as usual

2. I have looked forward with enjoyment to things No, I have been coping as well as ever

As much as I ever did

Rather less than I used to *7 I have been so unhappy that I have had difficulty sleeping

Definitely less than I used to Yes, most of the time

Hardly at all Yes, sometimes

Not very often

*3. I have blamed myself unnecessarily when things No, not at all

went wrong

Yes, most of the time *8 I have felt sad or miserable

Yes, some of the time Yes, most of the time

Not very often Yes, quite often

No, never Not very often

No, not at all

4. I have been anxious or worried for no good reason

No, not at all *9 I have been so unhappy that I have been crying

Hardly ever Yes, most of the time

Yes, sometimes Yes, quite often

Yes, very often Only occasionally

No, never

*5 I have felt scared or panicky for no very good reason

Yes, quite a lot *10 The thought of harming myself has occurred to me

Yes, sometimes Yes, quite often

No, not much Sometimes

No, not at all Hardly ever

Never

Administered/Reviewed by _____ Date

---

1 Source: Cox, J.L., Holden, J.M., and Sagovsky, R. 1987. Detection of postnatal depression: Development of the 10-item
Edinburgh Postnatal Depression Scale. British Journal of Psychiatry 150:782-786 .
2 Source: K. L. Wisner, B. L. Parry, C. M. Piontek, Postpartum Depression N Engl J Med vol. 347, No 3, July 18, 2002,
194-199

Users may reproduce the scale without further permission providing they respect copyright by quoting the names of the

authors, the title and the source of the paper in all reproduced copies.

No, most of the time I have coped quite well

Edinburgh Postnatal Depression Scale 1 (EPDS)

Postpartum depression is the most common complication of childbearing. 2 The 10-question Edinburgh

Postnatal Depression Scale (EPDS) is a valuable and efficient way of identifying patients at risk for "perinatal"

depression. The EPDS is easy to administer and has proven to be an effective screening tool.

Mothers who score above 13 are likely to be suffering from a depressive illness of varying severity. The EPDS

score should not override clinical judgment. A careful clinical assessment should be carried out to confirm the

diagnosis. The scale indicates how the mother has felt **during the previous week.** In doubtful cases it may

be useful to repeat the tool after 2 weeks. The scale will not detect mothers with anxiety neuroses, phobias or

personality disorders.

Women with postpartum depression need not feel alone. They may find useful information on the web sites of

the National Women's Health Information Center <www.4women.gov> and from groups such as Postpartum

Support International <www.chss.iup.edu/postpartum> and Depression after Delivery
<www.depressionafterdelivery.com>.

SCORING

QUESTIONS 1, 2, & 4 (without an *)

Are scored 0, 1, 2 or 3 with top box scored as 0 and the bottom box scored as 3.

QUESTIONS 3, 510

(marked with an *)

Are reverse scored, with the top box scored as a 3 and the bottom box scored as 0.

Maximum score: 30

Possible Depression: 10 or greater

Always look at item 10 (suicidal thoughts)

Users may reproduce the scale without further permission, providing they respect copyright by quoting the

names of the authors, the title, and the source of the paper in all reproduced copies.

Instructions for using the Edinburgh Postnatal Depression Scale:

1. The mother is asked to check the response that comes closest to how she has been feeling
in the previous 7 days.

2. All the items must be completed.

3. Care should be taken to avoid the possibility of the mother discussing her answers with
others. (Answers come from the mother or pregnant woman.)

4. The mother should complete the scale herself, unless she has limited English or has difficulty
with reading.

1 Source: Cox, J.L., Holden, J.M., and Sagovsky, R. 1987. Detection of postnatal depression: Development of the 10-item
Edinburgh Postnatal Depression Scale. British Journal of Psychiatry 150:782-786.
2 Source: K. L. Wisner, B. L. Parry, C. M. Piontek, Postpartum Depression N Engl J Med

vol. 347, No 3, July 18, 2002,
194-199

REMEMBER TO DIAL 911 IF YOU ARE HAVING AN EMERGENCY

Following is a list of postpartum depression treatment programs, therapists, social workers, psychiatrists, psychologists and other specialists who help women with postpartum mood and anxiety disorders including postpartum depression, postpartum anxiety, postpartum OCD, postpartum psychosis and depression during pregnancy in the USA and Canada and a few International locations. Thank you to all those wonderful resources who contributed to making this collection. Any information in this resource may be copied and shared. We welcome the addition of more resources you know about, and also any updates or corrections to the information we were able to gather.

This list does not endorse any specific treatment program or healthcare provider, but may help you find local healthcare providers in your area who specialize in postpartum depression treatment and women's mental health.

If you want to add a name to this list or provide any feedback, please email the author at MaggieReese[at]NewIdeasPublishing[dot]com.

Alabama Postpartum Depression Treatment

Dothan – Lauren Spooner PhD

Dothan – Sarah Foy MEd, Alta Care

Montgomery – Family Guidance Center

Alaska Postpartum Depression Treatment

Anchorage – Providence Hospital Postpartum Support

Anchorage – Anchorage Women's Clinic, Paula Phillips LPC

Anchorage – Meghan Yarmak LPC

Fairbanks – Kinship Counseling

Kenai Peninsula – Hope Mends

Arkansas Postpartum Depression Treatment

Fayetteville – Ryan Davis LCSW

Fayetteville – Adriana Stacey MD

Little Rock – UAMS Mental Health Services for Pregnant & Postpartum Women

Arizona Postpartum Depression Treatment

Gilbert – Michelle Lacey MA

Gilbert – Ann-Marie Casey PMHNP

Mesa – Marianne Arcari Rubin, LCSW 480-380-6248

Scottsdale – Saba Mansoor MD

Tempe – Cara English MA, LAC, DBH

Tuscon – Univ of Arizona Perinatal Psychiatry Clinic

California Postpartum Depression Treatment

Belmont – Jacki Silber LMFT

Berkeley – Gina Hassan PhD

Berkeley – Phyllis Klaus MFT LCSW

Beverly Hills – Jessica Zucker PhD

Beverly Hills – Sherry Nafeh LMFT

Chico – Dona Templeman MFT

Claremont – Katayune Kaeni, Psy.D.

Culver City – Caitlin Tonda MFT

Cupertino – MFB Counseling

Cupertino – Pec Indman EdD MFT

Encino – Dalia Kenig MFT

Fresno – Nurture 2 Nurture

Kensington – Lee Safran, MFT

La Canada Flintridge – Ann Dypiangco LCSW

Lafayette – Meri Levy MA

Lafayette – Kimberly Kerlin MA

Lafayette – Emily Margalit MFT

Lafayette – Mt. Diablo Perinatal Psychotherapy Associates **(offices in both Lafayette and Mt Diablo)**

Long Beach – Community Hospital Long Beach Perinatal Mood and Anxiety Disorders Program **(inpatient and outpatient)**

Long Beach – Vivien Burt MD

Long Beach – Rose Hanna MS, LMFT

Long Beach CA, Community Hospital Long Beach Inpatient Program

Los Altos – Beryl Hattori PhD

Los Angeles – UCLA Women's Life Center Los Angeles

Los Angeles – Robin Harpster MA

Los Angeles – Dalia Kennig, **MFT**

Los Angeles – Jennifer Yashari MD

Los Angeles area (several locations) – Bienvenidos

Los Angeles – Great Beginnings for Black Babies

Los Angeles – Stephanie Zisook MD

Los Angeles – Well Baby Center

Los Angeles – Venice Family Clinic

Los Angeles – Terry Wohlberg, MA, LMFT

Los Angeles area – Maternal Mental Health Now Directory of Perinatal Mental Health Resources

Los Gatos – Michelle Cherry LMFT

Los Gatos – Dolat Bolandi MFT

Mar Vista – Well Baby Center

Monterey – Meg Grundy LCSW

Monterey- Jennifer Golden LCSW

Mountain View – El Camino Hospital Maternal Outreach Mood Services **(MOMS)**

Mt. Diablo – Mt. Diablo Perinatal Psychotherapy Associates

Newport Beach/Long Beach – Laura Navarro Pickens LCSW

Newport Beach – Alexis Meshi MD

Newport Beach – Genevieve Yu MD

Newport Beach – Sonya Rasminsky MD

Oakland – Miriam Shultz MD

Oakland – Donna Rothert PhD

Oakland – Rachel Tucker MFT

Orange County – Elizabeth Farnsworth LMFT

Orange County – St. Joseph's Hospital Caring for Women with Maternal Depression program

Orange County – Orange Co. Postpartum Wellness Program

Orinda – Katherine Shulz LCSW

Palo Alto – Elizabeth Eastman LCSW

Pasadena – The Maternal Wellness Program at Huntington Hospital

Pasadena – Emily Dossett, MD

Redondo Beach – Mother Nurture Center, Stephanie Morales MFT

Riverside – Emilia Ortega-Jara LCSW

Roseville – Lindsey Plumer LMFT

Roseville – Katie Read MFT

Sacramento – Catherine O'Brien

San Diego – UC San Diego Maternal Mental Health Program

San Diego - Yvonne Rothermel LCSW

San Diego – Abigail Burd LCSW

San Diego – Leslie Craig MD

San Diego – Gretchen Mallios LCSW

San Dimas – Andrea Schneider LCSW

for more specialized providers in San Diego, visit the Postpartum Health Alliance of San Diego provider list

San Francisco – Kaiser Permanente San Francisco, Chris Eaton, MD and Kerry Savola-Levin, LCSW, 415-833-2292

San Francisco — UC San Francisco WomenCare Mental Health Program

San Francisco – Sutter Health Perinatal Treatment Program

San Francisco – Perinatal Psychotherapy Services

San Francisco – Joanna Foote Adler PsyD

San Francisco – Juli Fraga PsyD

San Francisco – Renee Spencer LMFT

San Francisco – Kimberlee Sorem MD

San Francisco – San Francisco Counseling Group

San Francisco – Uma Lerner MD

San Francisco- Susan Allen, LMFT

San Francisco- Lila Aguilar Postpartum Doula

San Jose – Jessica Sorci, LMFT

San Jose – Angela Jensen-Ramirez LCSW

San Mateo – Cindy Donis MFT

Santa Clarita – Child Family Center

Santa Cruz – Amanda Fargo PsyD

Santa Barbara – Jan Broderick LCSW

Santa Barbara – Jenn Paul MFT

Santa Monica – Kelly Foster MD

Sebastopol – Tina Stanley LCSW

Sherman Oaks – Kira Stein

Sherman Oaks – Kristen Baird Goldman MA

Signal Hill – Transitions in Motherhood

Stanford – Stanford Women's Wellness Clinic

Tarzana – The Center for Postpartum Health

Torrance – Vi Ballard MA MFT

Torrance- Kitty Cleary Adamovic MS, LMFT, RN

Walnut Creek – Devlin Kelly PhD

Walnut Creek – Emily Margalit MFT

Whittier – Marisela Rosales LCSW

If you are seeking therapy offering a sliding scale fee based on income, or free counseling services, you might try the following:

Asian Community Mental Health Services **(Oakland)**, Center for the Pacific Asian Family **(LA)**, Casa de la Familia **(LA)**, Open Paths **(LA area)**, YOLO Family **(Davis, Woodland, West Sacramento)**

Colorado Postpartum Depression Treatment

Aurora – Children's Hospital Healthy Expectations Program, 303-864-5252

Boulder – Postpartum Wellness Center

Boulder – Kendra Miguez

Boulder – Nurturing Strategies LLC

Centennial – Kerri Langer, MD

Colorado Springs – Aimee Solis

Colorado Springs – Melissa Bannerot LMSW

Denver – Perinatal Mental Health Program at The Children's Hospital

Denver – Kym Thompson PsyD

Denver – Nancy Goodman LCSW

Denver – Bloom Health & Wellness, Jennifer Harned Adams PhD

Denver – Julie Gladnick, MA, LMFT

Denver – Michelle Luiz, Yao Clinic

Denver- Katie Godfrey PhD

Durango – Liv MacKenzie MA LPC

Fort Collins – Cherie Worford MD

Fort Collins – Holly Carpenter, MA

Lafayette– Jessica Hanlin, LCSW or 303-835-3552

Littleton – Mary Anderson Schroeter MSW

if you are seeking therapy offering a sliding scale fee based on income, or free counseling services, you might try the following: El Centro de las Familias (**Denver**), Wellshire Behavioral Services (**Denver**), Servicios de la Raza (**Denver**)

Connecticut Postpartum Depression Treatment

New Canaan – Emily Farnum LCSW

New Haven – Yale Medical Group

Old Greenwich – Carla Pileggi Caviola LPC

West Hartford – Sharon Thomason PhD, Laurie Silverman MSW

Westport – The Center for Postpartum Support

Westport – Christie Chapman LCSW

Delaware Postpartum Depression Treatment

Dover – Amy Didden LCSW

Newark – Aimee McFarlan, LCSW, Mid-Atlantic Behavioral Healthcare

Newark – Nikki Stryker LCSW

Wilmington – Christiana Care Center for Women's Emotional Wellness

Florida Postpartum Depression Treatment

Boca Raton – Laura Krieger LCSW

Boca Raton- Dr. Brandi Baumkirchner 561-404-9675

Boca Raton – Brian Schaflin

Ft. Lauderdale – Elizabeth Bonet PhD LMHC

Ft. Lauderdale – Noreen Commella, PSY.D., 954-873-8257

Gainesville – University of Florida, Jacqueline Hobbs MD

Gainesville – Lauren W. DePaola, LCSW, 352-278-2538

Gainesville – Melissa Mamatas LMHC, 352-262-7889

Hallandale Beach – Marcia Starkman MSN

Melbourne – Ascend Counseling, Suna Clinchard LMFT

Miami – Happy Start Counseling Services

Miami– Shelly Orlowsky PsyD

Miami – U of Miami Psychiatry, Women's Mental Health, 305-243-6400 (Dr. Jeffrey Newport)

North Palm Beach – Jennifer Hume LMHC

North Palm Beach – Kathryn Friedman LMHC 561-346-7152

North Palm Beach – Susan Tinsley, MA, LMFT 561-252-1871

Orlando – Shari-ann H. James, Ph.D. shariannj@gmail.com or (407) 451-4077

Orlando – Morgan Rahimi LMFT

Palm Beach Gardens – Jennifer Goldin, PhD 561-371-9522

Palm Beach Gardens – Jamie Wintz, LMHC

Sarasota – Forty Carrots Family Center

Tampa – Robin Maier LCSW

Tampa – Brittany Bevilacqua PhD

Tampa – Susan Posada PhD

If you are seeking therapy offering a sliding scale fee based on income, or free counseling services, you might try The Women's Center (Jacksonville)

Georgia Postpartum Depression Treatment

Athens – Shannen Malutinok

Atlanta – Emory Women's Mental Health Program

Atlanta – Kate Ferguson LPC

Atlanta – Licia Freeman MA

Atlanta – Sarah Hightower LAPC

Atlanta – Elizabeth O'Brien LPC

Lawerenceville – Peyton Rhodes Knight LAPC

Roswell – Natasha Thomas MD

Roswell – Shubha Swamy LPC

Marietta – Jacqueline Cohen LPC

for more PPD specialists in Georgia, visit the MHA of GA provider list if you are seeking therapy offering a sliding scale fee based on income, or free counseling services, you might try the following:

CETPA (Gwinnett County, focused on services for Latinos)

Idaho Postpartum Depression Treatment

Boise – Transitions Counseling, Torri Lockman MSW

Pocatello – Nicki Aubuchon Endsley PhD

if you are seeking therapy offering a sliding scale fee based on income, or free counseling services, you might try Community Outreach Counseling which offers support in various Idaho cities

Illinois Postpartum Depression Treatment

Champaign/Urbana – Crisis Nursery's Beyond Blue Program

Chicago & Skokie – Wellsprings Health

Chicago – Healthcare Alternative Systems

Chicago – Wildflower Center for Emotional Health

Chicago – Women's Mental Health Program, Loyola University

Chicago – Women's Behavioral Health Program, Rush University Medical Center

Chicago – UI Hospital Women's Mental Health Program

Elk Grove Village – **Alexian Brothers Health System**, Perinatal Intensive Outpatient Program

Elmhurst – Kate Jensen, LPC, CAADC, CCTP

Evanston – Brooke Laufer PhD

Glenview – Kelly J Martin **at Courage to Connect Therapeutic Center**

Hoffman Estates – Alexian Brothers Pregnancy & Postpartum Mood Disorders Program

Hoffman Estates - AMITA Health Perinatal IOP at Alexian Brothers Women & Children's Hospital

Hoffman Estates – Postpartum Wellness Center

Lake Forest – Interchange Psychological Services

Lisle – Nina Appadurai PsyD

Naperville – Dawn Leprich-Graves, LPC

Naperville – Edward-Elmhurst Healthcare

Naperville – Naperville Clinical Associates, **Monica Schmitt PsyD**

Northbrook – Dr. Sarah Allen

Northbrook – Nikki Lively LCSW

Skokie – Susan Benjamin Feingold PsyD

Wheaton – Mary Jackson Lee LCSW

Wheaton – Fatima Ali MD

Wheaton – Sarah Cline LCSW

if you are seeking therapy offering a sliding scale fee based on income, or free counseling services, you might try: The Family Institute serving Evanston, Chicago, Northbrook and LaGrange or the Chicago Women's Health Center, or Community Health, or Courage to Connect Therapeutic Center in Glenview

Indiana Postpartum Depression Treatment

Carmel – Indiana Health Group, Amy Ricke MD

Indianapolis — Indiana University Specialized Women's Care

West Lafayette – **Calla Counseling,** Simone Yoemans PhD

Iowa Postpartum Depression Treatment

Ames – Central Iowa Psychological Services

Cedar Rapids – Shannon Wilson LMHC

Des Moines – Unity Point, **Donna Richard Langer**

Iowa City – University of Iowa Women's Wellness & Counseling Service

Pella – Pine Rest Pella Clinic, **Jill Thomas, LISW**

Urbandale – **Jill Thomas, LISW 515-331-0303**

Waterloo – Covenant Midwives & Women's Health Center

West Des Moines – Central Iowa Psychological Services (Karin Beschen, **LMHC, specializing in postpartum mental health**)

Kansas Postpartum Depression Treatment

Overland Park – Tonya Miles PsyD

Overland Park – Suzanne Heffner LCMFT

Prairie Village – Meeka Centimano

Wichita – Sarah Post LSCSW

Kentucky Postpartum Depression Treatment

Lexington – Colby Cohen Archer PhD

Louisville – Norton Women's Counseling, **Amanda Hettinger and Michelle Walden**

for more PPD specialists in Kentucky, visit the Postpartum Support Kentuckiana provider list

Louisiana Postpartum Depression Treatment

Baton Rouge – Cathy Gaston LCSW

Baton Rouge – **Woman's Hospital,** Renee Bruno MD

Baton Rouge – Eva Mathews MD

New Orleans – Kendall Genre MD

New Orleans – Dana Labat PhD

Shreveport – Center for Families

if you are seeking therapy offering a sliding scale fee based on income, or free counseling services, you might try the Children's Bureau of New Orleans

Maine Postpartum Depression Treatment

Portland – Martha Barry PhD

South Portland – Jenna Daly, LCSW

Maryland Postpartum Depression Treatment

Baltimore – Jennifer Teitelbaum Palmer MD

Baltimore – LifeBridge Health Perinatal Depression Outreach Program **Contact: Sara Daly, LCSW-C** (410) 601-7832

Ellicott City – Anne Waller, LCSW

Greenbelt – Courtney Marshall PMHNP

Hagerstown – Jenna Taylor LCPC

Lutherville – Safiyyah Abdul-Rahman MD

Lutherville – Alison L. Miller, Psy.D. and Associates

Montgomery County only- Aspire Counseling: Perinatal Depression-Healthy Mothers, Healthy Babies Program **Contact: America Caballero, LCPC** (301) 978-9750

Olney – Lisa Garcia LCSW

for more specialized PMH Providers, Programs, and Support Groups in Maryland, visit the DMV PMH Resource Guide

if you are seeking therapy offering a sliding scale fee based on income, or free counseling services, you might try The Pro Bono Project **which offers free counseling in MD**

Massachusetts Postpartum Depression Treatment

Boston – Massachusetts General Hospital's Center for Women's Mental Health

Boston – Brigham and Women's Hospital Women's Mental Health Program

Boston – **Tufts,** Judith Robinson MD **and** Vivian Halfin MD

Cambridge – Laurie Ganberg LICSW

Cambridge – Suzan Wolpow LMHC

Lexington – **Ellen Hilsinger MD, 781-863-5225**

Roslindale – The Leggett Group

Somerville – Vicky Reichert LMHC

Wakefield – Janice Goodman

Waltham – Jewish Family & Children's Services PPD Support

Waltham – Jessica Foley MA

Watertown – Mara Acel Green LICSW

Wellesley Hills – Deborah Issokson PsyD

Westborough – Carolyn Chapman MSW

Worcester – University of Massachusetts Medical School Women's Mental Health Program

Worcester – Birchtree Psychology, Rachel Smook PsyD

for more PPD specialists in Massachusetts, visit the North Shore PPD Task Force's provider list

if you are seeking therapy offering a sliding scale fee based on income, or free counseling services, you might try: La Alianza (Boston, Roxbury)

Michigan Postpartum Depression Treatment

Ann Arbor – University of Michigan Women & Infants Mental Health Program

Ann Arbor – St. Joseph Mercy Women's Mental Health Program

Ann Arbor – Valerie Wood LMSW

Birmingham – Camille Greenwald PhD

Birmingham – Dr. Howard Belkin

Bloomfield Hills – Laura Fadell PhD

Bloomfield Hills – Amanda Kopp PsyD

Bloomfield Hills – Ann Smith PsyD

Brighton – Kayla Katterman MA

Cadillac – Sydnie Simmons PsyD

Douglas – Kim Richardson

Farmington Hills – Lifestart Counseling, Marina Pesserl

Farmington Hills – Miriam Zuroff PhD

Grand Rapids — Pine Rest Mother and Baby Program

Highland – Antoinette Peterson MSW

Holland/Wyoming – Remi Spicer LMSW

Lansing – Jennifer Novello

Oakland County – Lisa Kruman LMSW

Petoskey – Joelle Drader MD

Rochester Hills — Roots & Wings Counseling

Royal Oak/Troy — Beaumont Children's Hospital Parenting Program

Troy – Varsha Karamchandani MD

Utica – Laura Espinosa PsyD

West Bloomfield – Rachel Zager LMSW

West Bloomfield – Lori Jacobs, **MA, LPC**

if you are seeking therapy offering a sliding scale fee based on income, or free counseling services, you might try: Univ. of Detroit Mercy Counseling Clinic

Minnesota Postpartum Depression Treatment

Eagan – Hatch Life

Eagan – Stages Counseling

Edina – Flourish Counseling

Maple Grove – Sara Biewen MA

Minneapolis – Hennepin Women's Mental Health Program (Outpatient)

Minneapolis – Hennepin County Medical Center Mother-Baby Program (Intensive Outpatient)
Hennepin Mother-Baby Day Hospital

Minneapolis, St. Paul & Edina – The Postpartum Counseling Center

Minneapolis – Laura Barbeau LMFT

Minneapolis – Jess Helle Morrissey MSW

Minneapolis – Dwenda Gjerdingen MD, Univ of Minnesota Bethesda Clinic

Minneapolis – Pam Cleary LICSW

Minneapolis/St. Paul – Mother Baby Center

St. Cloud – St. Cloud Hospital Women's Behavioral Health Clinic

St. Louis Park – Andrea Szporn PhD

St. Paul – Shoshana Center for Reproductive Health Psychiatry

St. Paul – Suzanne Swanson PhD

St. Paul – Dr. Jeanette Truchsess Phd

for more Minnesota providers, visit http://ppsupportmn.org/

if you are seeking therapy offering a sliding scale fee based on income, or free counseling services, you might try the Walk-In Clinic **(Minneapolis)**

Missouri Postpartum Depression Treatment

Columbia – Erica Kroll LPC

Gladstone – Debra Mossinghoff MD

St. Louis – Elizabeth Lowder LCSW

St. Louis – Midwest Mind Body Health Center, Diane Sanford PsyD

St. Louis – Sarah Coffman MSW

St. Louis – Robin Androphy MD at The Counseling Center

St. Louis – St. Louis Doulas (Postpartum Doula services)

St. Louis- Center for Counseling and Family Therapy

if you are seeking therapy offering a sliding scale fee based on income, or free counseling services, you might try the Family Resource Center (St. Louis)

Montana Postpartum Depression Treatment

Billings – Karen Keitzman PsyD

Bozeman – Kate Robinett MSW

Bozeman- Jennifer Viciedo MS LCPC

Missoula – Jennifer Walrod LCSW

Nebraska Postpartum Depression Treatment

Omaha – Methodist Women's Counseling Program

Papillion – Kristen Treat, LMHP

Nevada Postpartum Depression Treatment

Las Vegas – Dena Johns

New Hampshire Postpartum Depression Treatment

Manchester (and other locations) – Child & Family Services

Windham – Perinatal & Women's Mental Health Counseling

New Jersey Postpartum Depression Treatment

Chatham — Laura Winters LCSW

Cherry Hill — Meridian Counseling

Cranford – Michael Barmak LCSW

Elmer and Sewell – Kate DeStefano-Torres

Hoboken – Linda Chuang, MD

Livingston – Beth Sonnenberg LCSW

Longbranch – Monmouth Medical Center Perinatal Mood & Anxiety Program

Long Beach Island (Brant Beach)- St. Francis Community Center Counseling

Shrewsbury – Integrative Psychotherapy, Kristen M Levitt LCSW

Summit – Rosalind Dorlen, PsyD

Summit- Jennifer Bronswick, MSW

Tenafly – Blue Sky Consulting LLC

Tinton Falls – Birth, Babies & Beyond

Turnersville – The Postpartum Stress Center

Waldwick – The Women's Wellness Center of Bergen County

Wayne – Kathy Morelli LPC

New Mexico Postpartum Depression Treatment

Albuquerque – Wallin & Luna

Las Cruces – Andrea Dresser LMFT

Santa Fe – Kate Dow PhD

New York Postpartum Depression Treatment

Brooklyn – Sparks Center

Brooklyn/Manhattan – Emma Basch PsyD

Brooklyn/Manhattan – Jennifer Rhodes MD

Brooklyn – Flora Margolis LCSW

Brooklyn – Ellen Krug LCSW

Buffalo – Jennifer Urban LCSW-R

Carmel – Sinead Macnamara-Murphy LCSW

Croton-on-Hudson – Agathe Pierre-Louis PsyD

East Setauket – Passages Wellness for Women

Garden City – Cheryl Zauderer PhD

Glen Oaks, Queens County NY, Northwell Health Perinatal Psychiatry Service

Kingston – Liz Fernandez LCSW

Manhattan – Carly Snyder MD

Manhattan – Payne Whitney Women's Program at Weill Cornell, New York

Manhattan – New York University Reproductive Psychiatry, New York

Manhattan – Alexandra Sacks MD

Manhattan – Dr. Kira Bartlett, PsyD

Manhattan – Women's Mental Health Consortium, New York

Manhattan – Seleni Institute

Manhattan – Columbia University Psychiatry Women's Program

Manhattan – Sabrina Khan, MD

Manhattan (Upper East Side) – Kathleen Rein MD

Manhattan - The Motherhood Center of New York

Manhattan – Parenthood Psychology Practice

Manhattan – Erika Cooley LCSW

Manhattan (Central Park West) – Laura Polania MD

Manhattan – Samantha Winokur PsyD

Manhattan (Union Square)/Brooklyn – Mommy Groove Therapy

Manhattan (Midtown, Chelsea) – Amanda Itzkoff MD

New York – Union Square Practice, Lucy Hutner,

Queens, Nassau and Suffolk Counties NY. Perinatal Psychiatry Services at The Zucker Hillside Hospital and South Oaks Hospital

Mt. Kisco – Susan Goodman MD

Rochester – Nicole Crump LMSW

Rochester – Linda Chaudron MD

Rochester – University of Rochester Perinatal Consultation Clinic

Rochester – Alexa Weeks **LMSW, RN-CLC, CD**

Westchester – Kira Bartlett PsyD

for more PPD specialists throughout NY state, visit the Postpartum Resource Center of New York provider list if you are seeking therapy offering a sliding scale fee based on income, or free counseling services, you might try the Child Center of NY (Flushing, Jamaica and Woodside), or the Steinway Child & Family Services (Long Island)

North Carolina Postpartum Depression Treatment

Apex – Lifescapes Counseling

Chapel Hill – University of North Carolina Center for Women's Mood Disorders, Chapel Hill

Chapel Hill - UNC Perinatal Psych Inpatient Unit

Chapel Hill – Nicola Gray MD

Chapel Hill – Carolina Wellness Psychiatry

Charlotte – The Prenatal and Postpartum Center of the Carolinas

Fayetteville – Beth Barrington LPCA

Matthews – Rachel Matthew, LCSW

Raleigh – Betty Shannon Prevatt LPA

Raleigh – Dori Pelz Sherman PhD

Raleigh – Margot Holloman

Winston Salem – Katherine Dawson Atala MD

if you are seeking therapy offering a sliding scale fee based on income, or free counseling services, you might try MHA Triangle (Durham, Orange, Person & Chatham Counties)

North Dakota Postpartum Depression Treatment

Devils Lake – Dr. Sara Kenney

Ohio Postpartum Depression Treatment

Beachwood – Allison Snyer PhD

Cincinnati – UC Psychiatry at the Women's Center

Cleveland – Cleveland Clinic Reproductive Psychiatry

Cleveland – Women's Mental Health Program at University Hospitals of Cleveland, Case Western Reserve University School of Medicine

Cleveland – Ohio Guidestone **(includes home-based counseling services)**

Columbus – OSU Women's Behavioral Health Program **Dr. Julie Hyman**

Mason – Lindner Center of Hope Women's Mental Health Program

Worthington – Dawn Friedman LPC

if you are seeking therapy offering a sliding scale fee based on income, or free counseling services, you might try: the Centers for Families & Children (Cleveland), Womanline (Dayton area)

Oklahoma Postpartum Depression Treatment

Edmond – Tara Fritsch LCSW

Moore – Balance Women's Health

Oklahoma City – Aimee Benton

if you are seeking therapy offering a sliding scale fee based on income, or free counseling services, you might try the following: Family & Children's Services (Tulsa)

Oregon Postpartum Depression Treatment

Beaverton – Wildwood Psychiatric Resource Center

Bend – Kim Martin LPC

Corvallis/Eugene – Csilla Andor LCSW

Eugene – Natalie Berkman LCSW

Medford – Megan Stonelake, MA, QMHP, 541-774-3870

Portland – Oregon Health & Science University Perinatal Mental Health Program, **Nicole Cirino MD**

Portland – Beth Bassett

Portland – Nurture Counseling Services

Portland – Sarah Baird PsyD

Portland – Motheroots Counseling

Portland – Megan Furnish MSW LCSW

for more specialists in Oregon, visit the Baby Blues Connection local provider list

Pennsylvania Postpartum Depression Treatment

Abington – Kellie Wicklund LPC

Bethlehem – Jennifer Perreault

Blakely – Maternal Mental Health & Wellness of Northeast PA

Bucks County – Melissa Hubsher PsyD

Bryn Mawr – Dr. Carly Goldberg

Camp Hill – Holy Spirit Healthcare Women's Behavioral Health

Carlisle – Judith DeRicco LPC

Carlisle- Valerie Domenici PhD

Chester/Upland – Crozer Keystone Perinatal Mental Health Program

Doylestown – Shanthi Trettin MD

Greensburg – Brittany Edge MA LMFT

Lancaster – Women & Babies Hospital Women's Behavior Health Counseling

Lancaster/York – Pressley Ridge

Lancaster – Laurie Vogt LMFT

New Kensington – Emotional Wellness for Her

Newtown Square – Main Line Health Women's Emotional Wellness Center

Newtown – Christine Haas PhD

Philadelphia – Penn Center for Women's Behavioral Wellness

Philadelphia -- Drexel University Mother Baby Connections Intensive Outpatient Program

Philadelphia – The Center for Postpartum Depression

Philadelphia – Women's Mental Health Associates

Philadelphia – Perri Shaw Borish LCSW

Philadelphia – Alisa Kamis-Brinda, LCSW, LCADC

Philadelphia – "Alex" Caroline Robboy, CAS, MSW, LCSW

Pittsburgh – Magee Women's Behavioral Health Services

Women's Behavioral Health West Penn Hospital Allegheny Health Network

Pittsburgh – Amy Lewis LSW

Pittsburgh – Emotional Wellness for Her

Rosemont/Devon/Turnersville(NJ) – The Postpartum Stress Center

Scranton – Cara Koslow LPC

Sharon – Laura McElhinny LCSW

West Chester – Erin Saddic MS

if you are seeking therapy offering a sliding scale fee based on income, or free counseling services, you might try: Therapy Center of Philadelphia

Rhode Island Postpartum Depression Treatment

Pawtucket – Melissa Etting LCMHC

Providence – Women and Infants Hospital Day Program

Providence – Women's Behavioral Medicine

South Carolina Postpartum Depression Treatment

Charleston – Medical University of South Carolina Postpartum Mood Disorders Program

Charleston – Jessica Gregg

Columbia – Midlands Psychiatric, Stephanie Berg MD & Kelly Helms LISW

Greenville – Susannah Baldwin, MEd, LPCI

Lexington – Jill Smith Therapy

Mt. Pleasant – Beth Keyserling LMFT

Mt. Pleasant – Dr. Risa Byars in Mount Pleasant, 843-769-0444

Mt. Pleasant – East Cooper Psychiatric Associates

Mt. Pleasant – Beth Keyserling LMFT LPC

Summerville – Women's Health Partners (Kysten Sutton and Beth Cook), 843-832-5096

Tennessee Postpartum Depression Treatment

Memphis – Beth Shelton Hayes LMSW

Nashville – Dr. Margot Feintuch, 615-269-0525

Nashville – Hope Clinic for Women

Nashville – Ruth Bryant LMSW

Texas Postpartum Depression Treatment

Austin – for PPD specialists in the Austin area, visit the Pregnancy & Postpartum Health Alliance of Texas' provider list

Austin – Kelly Boyd PsyD

Austin – Counseling for New Moms

Austin – Jan Morris PhD

Cypress – Your Family Psychiatrist

Dallas – Women's Mental Wellness

Dallas – Parkland Hospital

Dallas – Kim Kertsburg, LCSW

Dallas – Christy Tucker, PhD

Dallas/Southlake – Neysa Johnson, MD

Dallas/Southlake – Anna Brandon PhD

Houston – The Women's Place, Texas Children's Hospital

Houston – Sherry Duson MA

Houston – Center for Postpartum Family Health

Houston – Galleria Counseling

Houston – Kristin Calverly, Ph.D.

Houston – Jacqueline Sim, LMFT

Kingwood – Deborah Olson

McKinney – Christina Spinler

San Antonio – Maria Zeitz

San Antonio – Sue Clifford LPC

The Woodlands – Irena Milentijevic

if you are seeking therapy offering a sliding scale fee based on income, or free counseling services, you might try:

Family Services of Greater Houston, Texas Woman's Counseling & Family Therapy Clinic (Denton), Family Service of El Paso, Family Support Services (Amarillo), the Family Place (Dallas)

Utah Postpartum Depression Treatment

Midvale – The Healing Group

Salt Lake City – Amy Rose White LCSW

Salt Lake City – Mandi Stevenson MA

Salt Lake City/Draper/Sandy – Regan Haight APRN

Springville – Tara Tulley LCSW

if you are seeking therapy offering a sliding scale fee based on income, or free counseling services, you might try: Family Support Center (Taylorsville)

Vermont Postpartum Depression Treatment

South Burlington – Emily Miller MA, LCHMC

Virginia Postpartum Depression Treatment

Alexandria – Evolve Clinical Services, Elizabeth Hatchuel PhD

Centreville – Beverly Reader MD

Fairfax – Terri Adams LCSW

Falls Church – Benta Sims

Norfolk – Christine Truman MD

Richmond – Linda Zaffram LCSW

note: for more specialized PMH Providers, Programs, and Support Groups in Virginia, visit Postpartum Support Virginia (PSVA)

If you are seeking therapy offering a sliding scale fee based on income, or free counseling services, try The Women's Initiative (Charlottesville)

Washington Postpartum Depression Treatment

Bellingham – Mobile Mama Therapy

Edmonds – Terri Buysse, Ph.D.

Issaquah – **Corey Hope Colwell-Lipson LMFT, 206-818-7591**

Kirkland – Renee Bibault MD

Kirkland – Heidi Koss LMHC

Lynnwood – LifeCircle Counseling and Consulting, LLC

Redmond – Lin Thoennes NP

Seattle – Swedish Perinatal Center for Perinatal Bonding and Support

Seattle – Jennifer Palermo

Seattle – Leslie Butterfield PhD

Seattle – Teresa Williams LICSW

Seattle – Sarah Palmer MA

Seattle – Christie Messina MA, LMHC

Seattle – **Patricia Spach, 206-522-3543**

Seattle – Shannon Armitage LMFT

Tacoma – Bloom

Tacoma – Virginia Buccola Tournay DNP

Tacoma – Anna Maria Sierra

Vancouver – Ann Walsleben MS

If you are seeking therapy offering a sliding scale fee based on income, or free counseling services, try the Seattle Therapy Alliance

Washington DC Postpartum Depression Treatment

George Washington University Women's Mental Health 5 Trimesters Clinic

MedStar Georgetown University Hospital Women's Mental Health Program & Perinatal Mental Health Clinic Contact: Aimee Danielson, PhD (202) 944-5412

Jennifer Kogan MSW

Emily Griffin MSW

Parker Kennedy Rea, PsyD

Lynne McIntyre MSW, info@postpartumdc.org or 202.643.7290

note: for more specialized PMH Providers, Programs, and Support Groups in DC, visit the DMV PMH Resource Guide

If you are seeking therapy offering a sliding scale fee based on income, or free counseling services, try DC Counseling Connection or The Women's Center

Wisconsin Postpartum Depression Treatment

Madison – Emily Barr Ruth PsyD

Madison – Jen Perfetti MA

Madison – Emily Hagenmeier LCSW

Mequon – Rose Eichenhofer LCSW

Milwaukee — Dr. Christina Wichman, **Medical College of Wisconsin**

Milwaukee – Abby Kruyper PsyD

Wauwatosa – Kathryn Vele MSN, APNP

If you are seeking therapy offering a sliding scale fee based on income, or free counseling services, try Children's Hospital of Wisconsin's Child & Family Therapy, offered in Eau Claire, Kenosha, Madison, Milwaukee, Racine, Stevens Point and more

INTERNATIONAL RESOURCES

http://www.nlm.nih.gov/medlineplus/languages/postpartumdepressio n.html

Postpartum Depression Information in 15 languages, included Arabic, Japanese, Korean, Chinese, Vietnamese, Russian and Somali

French: Societe Marce Francophone
http://www.marce-francophone.fr/

German
http://www.marce-gesellschaft.de/

Hebrew

http://www.health.gov.il/Subjects/pregnancy/Childbirth/birthday/ Pages/postnatal_depressions.aspx

http://www.health.gov.il/PublicationsFiles/Postnatal_depression.p df

University of California, San Francisco, Depression Prevention Course (Muñoz)

http://medschool2.ucsf.edu/latino/pdf/mothers_babiesES/mbpclas
s1SP.pdf
Workbooks available in Spanish, Japanese, Chinese, English

Maternal & Child Health Library, Non-English Language
Resources
http://www.mchlibrary.info/nonenglish.html

Pacific Post Partum Support Society Resources

Simplified Chinese: http://postpartum.org/translations/chinese-
simplified/
Traditional Chinese: http://postpartum.org/translations/chinese-
traditional/
Farsi: http://postpartum.org/translations/farsi/
Punjabi: http://postpartum.org/translations/punjabi/
Spanish: http://postpartum.org/translations/spanish/

INTERNATIONAL

AUSTRALIA

Royal Women's Hospital Centre for Women's Mental Health,
Victoria

Mercy Hospital Perinatal Mental Health, Victoria

North Shore Private Hospital Emotional Wellbeing Program,
Sydney

Beyond Blue

COPE

PANDA: Post and Antenatal Depression Association

TABS: Trauma & Birth Stress

CANADA

Life With A Baby **(Ontario)**

Mother Reach **(London)**

Postpartum Mood Disorder Project Ontario

Moms Supporting Moms **(Milton area)**

Pacific Postpartum Support Society **(BC)**

Manitoba Postpartum Warm Line 204-391-5983 **(9am until 9pm)**

Postpartum Depression Awareness **(Kelowna, Edmonton)**

Postpartum Depression Association of Manitoba **(Manitoba)**

PPD Support Line **(Brantford, Ontario)**

Alberta Postpartum Depression Treatment

Foothills Medical Centre Women's Mental Health Clinic, **Calgary**

Birth Narratives – Shannon Kane, **Calgary**

Tamara Hanoski, PhD, **Edmonton**

The Family Centre, **Edmonton**

Claire Wilde R.Psych., **Edmonton**

British Columbia Postpartum Depression Treatment

Reproductive Mental Health Program at St. Paul's Hospital and BC Women's, **Vancouver**

Jim Pattison Outpatient Center, **Surrey**

Abbotsford Perinatal Depression Support

Ontario Postpartum Depression Treatment

Rebirth Wellness – Jodi Tiller MSW, **London**

Canadian Mental Health Association, **Oxford County**

NOVA Counseling, **Sudbury**

St. Clair Services, **Sarnia**

Michelle Lavergne, MSW, **Thornhill/York**

Eliana Cohen PhD, **Toronto**

Perinatal Mental Health Program at Mt. Sinai Hospital, **Toronto**

Women's College Hospital Women's Mental Health Program, **Toronto**

UHN Women's Mental Health, **Toronto**

Canadian Mental Health Association, **Woodstock**

Women's Health Concerns Clinic, **St. Joseph's Healthcare Hamilton**

Royal Ottawa Women's Mental Health Program, **Ottawa**

Trillium Women's Reproductive Health Program, **Mississauga**

Nova Scotia

IWK Reproductive Mental Health Services, **Nova Scotia**

IRELAND

Dublin – National Maternity Hospital Perinatal Mental Health

PND Ireland

SCOTLAND (UNITED KINGDOM)

Crossreach Postnatal Depression Lothian

Bluebell PND Glasgow

UNITED KINGDOM

The Association for Postnatal Illness

PANDAS (England & Wales)

PNI (Postnatal Illness) UK

Mums Aid (Greenwich)

Action Postpartum Psychosis

House of Light (Kingston upon Hull/East Riding)

Open House – Notts (**Nottingham**)

Sheffield Light

Acacia Postnatal Depression Support (Birmingham)

Joanne Bingley Memorial Foundation

Bluebell (Bristol)

Birth Trauma Association UK

UK Postnatal Depression Treatment

Beckhenham – Bethlem Royal Hospital Mother and Baby Unit

Birmingham — Birmingham Perinatal Mental Health Service Mother and Baby Unit

Bristol — Southmead Hospital New Horizon Mother Baby Unit

Chelmsford — Rainbow Mother Baby Unit

Glasgow — West of Scotland Mother and Baby Unit

Leeds — Leeds Mother & Baby Unit

Leicester — Bradgate Mother and Baby Unit

London — Coombe Wood Mother Baby Unit

Lothian – Crossreach

Manchester — Anderson Ward Mother & Baby Unit

Morpeth — Northumberland Mother and Baby Unit

Southampton – Southern Mother and Baby Unit

South London — Bethlem Royal Hospital Mother Baby Unit

Winchester — Winchester Mother and Baby Unit

NEW ZEALAND

- Need to talk? (1737 – free call or text)
- the Depression Helpline (0800 111 757)
- Lifeline (0800 543 354)
- the Samaritans (0800 726 666)
- Youth line (0800 376 633)
- Plunket (0800 933 922)
- the Mental Health Foundation of New Zealand

- the Postnatal Distress Support Network Trust.

PND New Zealand (Wellington)

Mothers Matter

SOUTH AFRICA

Postnatal Depression Support Association

Perinatal Mental Health Project

SWITZERLAND

HUG Child Counseling Unit – Nathalie Nanzer

Postpartum Depression Support Groups in the U.S. & Canada

Postpartum Depression Support Groups in the U.S. & Canada

Online Resources:

http://www.1800ppdmoms.org
http://www.apa.org/pi/women/resources/reports/postpartum-dep.aspx
http://www.postpartum.net 1.800.944.4773

Postpartum Depression HOPE Hotline –1-800-944-4PPD

ALABAMA POSTPARTUM DEPRESSION SUPPORT

Madison — Huntsville Postpartum Support Network, Hope Church 1661 Balch Road, Madison. Contact Teresa 703-622-0986 or at tkfleisch@gmail.com

ALASKA POSTPARTUM DEPRESSION SUPPORT

Anchorage — Monday Mama's Support group. Postpartum Support Alaska meets at the Maternity Education Center at the Children's Hospital at Providence. Contact the Family Support Counseling Clinic at 907-212-4940 or Joclyn Reilly, Family Support Services counselor.

Fairbanks – Alaska Family Health & Birth Center Support Group. Contact 907-456-3719 to register

ARIZONA POSTPARTUM DEPRESSION SUPPORT

Flagstaff — Postpartum Adjustment Support Group at North County Healthcare. Contact 928-707-0748 to register

Gilbert – Pregnancy and Postpartum Support Group at Dignity Health. Wednesdays from 1 to 2:30 p.m. (Support groups do not meet week of July 4th, Thanksgiving, Christmas and New Year's) **Free**. Moms may bring a support person with them. Infants and toddlers are welcome. Rome Towers, 1760 E Pecos Rd., #235 Gilbert, AZ 85295

Glendale — New Moms Postpartum Support Group meets at Banner Thunderbird Medical Center. Contact 602-865-5908

Mesa — Pregnancy and Postpartum Adjustment Support Group meets Tuesdays from 10-11:30 at Banner Desert Medical Center; contact 480-412-5292

Scottsdale — Pregnancy and Postpartum Depression Support Group Facilitated by a licensed psychologist (Dr. Abby Garcia) this group is for moms experiencing depression or anxiety during pregnancy or after childbirth. The group meets in the first floor conference room at the Virginia G. Piper Cancer Center on the Shea Medical Center campus. For more information, please call 480-323-3878. It meets the first and third Friday of every month. 9:30am-11:30am

Phoenix — Mother to Mother support group at St. Joseph's Hospital, Contact 1-877-602-4111

Tucson — Pregnancy and Postpartum Adjustment Support Group at Northwest Medical Center. Contact Alison at 520-877-4149

Tucson — Postpartum Depression Support Group at St. Joseph's Hospital. Contact Carole at 520-873-6858

You can also call the Arizona Postpartum Warmline at 1-888-434-MOMS

ARKANSAS POSTPARTUM DEPRESSION SUPPORT

Rogers- PPD Support Group. The Joshua Center 2105 S. 54th St. #2 Cost: $25 session. RSVP required. Contact Heidi at Heidi@thejoshuacenter.com

CALIFORNIA POSTPARTUM DEPRESSION SUPPORT

Auburn – Insights Counseling Group. 8207 Sierra College Blvd. Contact (530) 887-1300 or Colleen@insightscounselinggroup.org

Berkeley — North Berkeley Postpartum Stress Support Group. Contact Lee Safran at 510-496-6096

Beverly Hills — What about Mommy? A postpartum Group for Mothers, contact (310) 929-0638

Claremont — Postpartum support group. Email drkaeni@gmail.com or call 909-451-9951.

Clearlake — Mother-Wise. Contact Jaclyn at 707-349-1210 or visit our Facebook page for more event
information https://www.facebook.com/MotherWiseLakeCounty

Escondido – Moms in Bloom Call (760) 489-1092 or
email **inpsychcenter@gmail.com** to reserve your spot or get information. A free phone consultation will be provided for entrance to the group.

Fresno — Babies R Us. Facilitators: Stephanie Chandler, PM & Susan Kordell, RN. Contact 559-244-4580

Fresno — First 5 Lighthouse for Children 2405 Tulare St. Fresno, 93721. Facilitator: Alejandra Addo-Boateng, MFTI, 559-244-4580

La Jolla — at Scripps Memorial Hospital, call 1-800-SCRIPPS

La Mesa — at Sharp Grosmont Hospital, contact 619-740-4906

Lafayette – Postpartum Emotional Recovery Circle at Mt. Diablo Perinatal Psychotherapy Associates. Contact Meri Levy, MFT at 925-385-8848

Lakeport — Mother-Wise. Contact Jaclyn at 707-349-1210 or visit our Facebook page for more event
information https://www.facebook.com/MotherWiseLakeCounty

Long Beach — Transitioning Into Motherhood support services at Long Beach Memorial. Visit http://transitionsinmotherhood.com/events/

Los Gatos – Family Tree Wellness (click for schedule)

Los Gatos — El Camino Hospital Los Gatos Pregnancy & Postpartum Resiliency Circle; meets during the year in 6-week series; call for dates and times here 650-962-5745.

Madera — Fridays: 9-1030am, Family Resource Center, 525 E. Yosemite Ave. Madera, 93638. Facilitator: Roccio Arevalo, MFTI, bi-lingual English/Spanish, 559-675-4004

Monterey— Postpartum Support Groups. Contact 831-783-5933, email hello@parentingconnectionmc.org. Visit www.parentingconnectionmc.org

Mariposa —The Hub, 5078 Billion St. Mariposa. Facilitator: Jenny Morgan, 559-240-4370

Mission Viejo — Postpartum Adjustment Support Group at Mission Viejo Hospital. Contact Sue Harrison at 949-365-3818

Newport Beach — at Hoag Hospital. Contact Laura Navarro Pickens, LCSW for more information at (562) 882-7901

Oceanside — "Babies in Bloom". Contact Holly Herring, at 760-814-1421

Orange — at St. Joseph Hospital. Contact 714-771-8000 ext. 17891

Pacific Grove — Postpartum Wellness Support Group at Parent's Place. Contact Meg Grundy at 831-601-7021 or email meggrundy@yahoo.com

Pasadena – Motherhood Journey Therapy Groups for new and expectant mothers at the Institute for Girls' Development. Sonia Nikore, LMFT, 84145 at Institute for Girls Development at 626-585-8075 ext. 102

Pasadena – The Family Room. Contact Courtney at courtneyrachelnovak@gmail.com.

Roseville — PPD Support Group. Contact Kelly McGinnis at shineonsupport@outlook.com or 916-770-9394

San Diego — at Sharp Mary Birch Hospital. Contact 858-939-4141

San Francisco — Newborn Connections Postpartum Depression Support Group at California Pacific Medical Center, contact 415-600-2229

San Francisco — 6-week "Afterglow" PPD support group, held several times throughout the year, as part of UCSF Great Expectations Pregnancy program, for more info: http://www.whrc.ucsf.edu/whrc/gex/afterglow.html

San Francisco — Postpartum Support Groups led by Robyn Alagona

San Jose – Adjusting to Motherhood Emotional Support Group at Family Tree Wellness, Los Gatos. Contact Cheryl Hart (408) 475 4408 cheryl@supportingmamas.org

San Luis Obispo — Alpha Parenting PPD Support Line, 1-805-541-3367

San Luis Obispo — From a Pea to a Pumpkin prenatal support group. Tuesdays 3:15 – 4:30pm. Contact: (805)884-9794 or angela@angelawurtzelmft.com

Santa Barbara — From a Pea to a Pumpkin prenatal support group. Mondays 1:00 – 2:15pm. Contact: (805)884-9794 or angela@angelawurtzelmft.com

Serra Mesa — at Sharp Mary Birch Hospital. Contact 858-939-4141

Sherman Oaks – Motherhood Journey Postpartum Support Group at BINI Birth. Contact Robin Starkey Harpster, MA MFT rharpster@instituteforgirlsdevelopment.com 626-585-8075 ext. 109

Sherman Oaks – Postpartum Passages Contact Diana Barnes (818) 887-1312

COLORADO POSTPARTUM DEPRESSION SUPPORT

Boulder — Postpartum Transitions Group at the Postpartum Wellness Center. For more information and to register call 303-335-9473 or email rosie@pwcboulder.com.

Denver — PPD Support Group at Women's Therapy Center Cherry Creek. Contact Avery Neal at 866-995-7910

Denver – PPD Support at the Catalyst Center. For more information click here

Denver – Afterglow: Postpartum Therapy Group for Struggling Moms or Dads

Erie –Mothers Circle PPD support group at The Mother-Child Institute. Contact Rosie Falls, LCSW (303) 335-9473. Email rosie@motherchildinstitute.com. Web site: www.motherchildinstitute.com

Grand Junction — Western Slope Postpartum Peer Support Group,

Meets 1st and 3rd Saturdays 9:30am at Bloomin Babies Birth Center Meetings are free and include free childcare. Contact Emily Ridderman 970-901-7296

Littleton — Hope 4 Moms. Contact Mary Anderson Schroeter at 303-883-7271 or mary.schroeter@comcast.net. www.IntergrativePathwaysCounseling.com https://www.facebook.com/h4moms/

CONNECTICUT POSTPARTUM DEPRESSION SUPPORT

New Haven– Embracing Your Difference, Contact Venice Garner, LCSW 203-936-9213

Southport — Coastal Connecticut Counseling. Contact Jackie Small, MA, CLC – (203) 255-7480 ext.25 (203) 677-0891 www.jackiesmallma.com

Torrington – Charlotte Hungerford Hospital New Mother's Wellness Group, contact Amy Rodriguez at (860) 496-6359

West Hartford – Adjustment to Baby Challenges. Contact Annie Keating-Scherer at (860)212-7066 or Sharon Thomason at (860)331-1750

DELAWARE POSTPARTUM DEPRESSION SUPPORT

Newark, Wilmington & Dover — MOMs HEAL: Perinatal Mood Disorder Support Groups. Contact 302-733-6662 or email cwew@christianacare.org. http://www.christianacare.org/momsheal

FLORIDA POSTPARTUM DEPRESSION SUPPORT

Gainesville — Postpartum Adjustment Support Group

Gainesville — Postpartum Wellness & Family Counseling – 2 FREE groups: 2nd Wednesday monthly-5pm-6:30pm & 4th Monday monthly- 10am-11:30am (little ones welcome)

Ginesville — Postpartum Wellness & Family Counseling – Pregnancy and Infant Loss Support Group: 1st Sunday each month 2pm-3:30pm

Jacksonville — Baptist Health PPD Support Group

Orlando- Mothers Matter Support Group: Winnie Palmer Hospital call 321-841-5615

West Palm Beach- Circle of Moms Support Groups

Tampa – Coping with Motherhood PPD support group and Circle of Hope Group at St. Joseph's Women's Hospital. Call Kristina Davis at 813-872-3925.

GEORGIA POSTPARTUM DEPRESSION SUPPORT

Atlanta — Atlanta Postpartum Support Group, www.meetup.com/PPDAtlanta, meets monthly, contact Amber Koter at atlantamom930@gmail.com or call 914-261-8182

Carrollton – "Mommy's Day Out" Support Group. Contact Jwyanda Norman at 678-739-740 or email her at jwyanda@cloud.com

Dunwoody — PPD Support Group, contact cassieowenslpc@gmail.com or call 404-448-1733

Marietta — Emerge Into Light PPD support group.

You can also call the GA Project Healthy Moms Warmline for support at 1-800-933-9896 ext 234

HAWAII POSTPARTUM DEPRESSION SUPPORT

Oahu — PPD Support Group. Contact Diane at 808-392-7985

IDAHO POSTPARTUM DEPRESSION SUPPORT

Boise/Nampa — at St. Alphonsus Regional Medical Center, contact 208-367-7380

Ketchum — at the Center for Community Health. Contact 208-727-8733

Moscow — at Gritman Medical Center, contact 208-883-6385

ILLINOIS POSTPARTUM DEPRESSION SUPPORT

Chicago — Postpartum Depression Program at Healthcare Alternative Systems; Free services in English and Spanish. Call 773-292-4242

Chicago — Transitions to Motherhood program at Northwestern Memorial's Prentice Women's Hospital; Call 312-926-8400

Elk Grove – Door of Hope PPD support group at Alexian Brothers Medical Center; Call Lita Simanis at 847-981-3644 or lita.simanis@alexian.net

Elk Grove – La Maternidad y Yo: Spanish-language support group for new and expectant moms at Alexian Brothers Medical Center; call Natasha Varela at 847 755 8447 or Natasha.varela@alexian.net

Evanston — Beyond the Baby Blues PPD Support Group. Call 847-864-7957;

Glenview — Pregnancy and Postpartum Support Group at Courage to Connect. Call kelly@couragetoconnecttherapy.com or 847-730-3042

Hinsdale — PPD Support Group; call 630-856-4390.

Hoffman Estates — PPD support group. Call Lita Simanis at 847-755-3220

Hoffman Estates — MVP Men vs. Postpartum – Support group for fathers who have loved ones experiencing PPD; Call Lita Simanis at 847-755-3220

Moline/Quad Cities/Rock Island – Mothers Matter Support Groups

Northbrook – New Mom Support Group

Oak Lawn — Advocate Christ Conference Center. Call 708-684-1333

Oak Park — Parenthesis Parent Child Center, call Mary Strizak at 708-848-2227 or email mstrizak@parenthesis-info.org

Springfield—Postpartum Depression Support Group at HSHS St. John's Hospital—"New Moms Dealing with Feelings"; call the Parent Help Line (a toll-free confidential phone line) at 1-888-727-5889 or 1-217-544-5808 or email elizabeth.krah@hshs.org.

Winfield — Central DuPage Hospital. 630-933-1964

** For more Illinois support group information and resources, visit PPDIL

INDIANA POSTPARTUM DEPRESSION SUPPORT

Ft. Wayne — Lutheran Hospital support group, contact Michelle Dearmond, RN,BS, IBCLC at 260-435 7069 or mdearmond2@lutheran-hospital.com

Indianapolis — Indiana University Health, Contact Birdie Meyer at 317-962-8191 bmeyer2@iuhealth.org,

Indianapolis — Community Health Support group; Contact Marcia Boring MSW, LCSW, at 317-621-7828 or mboring@community.com

Indianapolis — Hendricks Regional Health support group; contact Brittany Waggoner, RN, BSN, CNS at 317-718-4018 or bswaggo@hendricks.org

Lafayette — Kathryn Weil Center support group; Contact 765-449-5133

South Bend — Mother Matters support group at South Bend Memorial Hospital, contact 574-647-3243 (or pager 574-236-7811, 8am-10pm)

South Bend — Peer support group for new moms at Good Shepherd Lutheran Church; Contact Linda Meeks at 574 272-3446

IOWA POSTPARTUM DEPRESSION SUPPORT

Bettendorf/Davenport – Mothers Matters Support Groups

Cedar Rapids — Murray, Wilson & Rose. Contact 319-213-6010

Des Moines – Pine Rest Des Moines Support Group, contact 515-331-0303

KANSAS POSTPARTUM DEPRESSION SUPPORT

Lawrence — at Lawrence Memorial Hospital (newborns welcome); Contact 785-505-3081 for more info

Overland Park —Contact the Postpartum Resource Center of Kansas at 913-677-1300

Shawnee Mission — Shawnee Mission Medical Center Postpartum Emotional Support Group

South Jackson County — Contact the Postpartum Resource Center of Kansas at 913-677-1300

Topeka – Sacred Circle of Northeast Kansas

KENTUCKY POSTPARTUM DEPRESSION SUPPORT

Lexington – The Postpartum Adjustment Center Contact 859-327-6459

For support you can also call the Postpartum Support Kentuckiana warmline at 502-541-1818

LOUISIANA POSTPARTUM DEPRESSION SUPPORT

Zachary – Lane Medical Center PPD Support Group, call 225-658-4587

MAINE POSTPARTUM DEPRESSION SUPPORT

Brunswick — PPD Support Group at Mid Coast Hospital, contact 207-373-6500 * Starting back up January 2016

MARYLAND POSTPARTUM DEPRESSION SUPPORT

Annapolis — at Anne Arundel Medical Center, Contact Ali Tiedke at 443-481-6124 or email atiedke@aahs.org

Baltimore — Postpartum Support Group at Sinai Hospital, contact Sara Daly, LCSW-C at 410-601-7832 or skdaly@lifebridgehealth.org

Elkton — Moms Matter Postpartum Support Group –Contact Beth Chipriano 410-620-3773 or bchipriano@uhcc.com.

Frederick County — Birthing Circle Contact thebirthingcircle@gmail.com

Leonardtown — (starting Jauary 18th, 2017) Empowered Connections – 10am-11am (for 6 weeks) (Wednesdays) Contact: Contact phone: 301-690-0779 Contact email: hello@empoweredconnections.net

Olney – Free weekly drop-in support group for pregnant and postpartum moms experiencing PMAD symptoms. For more info email: Anne Waller, LCSW-C aamcw@aol.com or Gina Keefe, APRN Ginakeefe@comcast.net

Silver Spring — PPD support group at Holy Cross Resource Center, free & no registration required, meets 1st and 3rd Sundays from 6-7:30pm; contact: MDpostpartum@gmail.com

MASSACHUSETTS POSTPARTUM DEPRESSION SUPPORT

Acton – Emotional Wellbeing After Baby group at First Connections, 179 Great Road, Suite 104; Contact Heather O'Brien hobrien@jri.org http://www.firstconnections.org/

Brookline – Support Group $25/session, Contact Rachel Kalvert, LICSW at 617-487-1521

Greenfield – Franklin County Postpartum Support Group at the Community Action Family Center, 90 Federal Street; Contact Sandy Clark at 413-475-1566, http://www.communityaction.us/

Plymouth – Depression After Delivery at Jordan Hospital, 275 Sandwich St., Meditation Room; Contact Gerri Piatelli at 781-837-4242, http://www.bidplymouth.org

Holyoke – MotherWoman Postpartum Support at Midwifery Care of Holyoke, 230 Maple Street, (413) 534 – 2700, http://www.motherwoman.org/

Waltham – "This Isn't What I Expected" PPD Support Group at JF&CS, 1430 Main Street; Contact Debbie Whitehill at 781-647-5327 x1925, dwhitehill@jfcsboston.org, http://www.jfcsboston.org/

North Reading – Postpartum Adjustment Support Groups at Stork Ready, 325 Mani Street; Contact Leslie McKeough at 781-507-2025, lamckeough@gmail.com, http://www.corevalu.com/

Newton – "Balance With Baby" Postpartum Support Group at The Freedman Center at William James College, One Wells Ave; Contact Chardae Golding at 617-332-3666 x 1123, Email: freedmancenter@williamjames.edu, http://www.williamjames.edu/community/freedman-center/index.cfm

Newton – Free Support Groups: http://www.williamjames.edu/community/freedman-center/new-moms.cfm

Watertown – Strong Roots PPD Support Groups, find information here.

MICHIGAN POSTPARTUM DEPRESSION SUPPORT

Bay City — Depression After Delivery Support Group, contact Sherry LaMere or Kelli Wilkinson at 989-895-2240

Clawson — Nature's Playhouse Traumatic Birth Support group, No registration necessary. Children are welcome. www.naturesplayhouse.com

Ferndale- Tree of Hope Support Group Call 586-372-6120 or email info@treeofhopefoundation.org.

Flint — PPD Support Group at Hurley Medical Center, no contact info available

Grand Haven — PPD Support Group at North Ottawa Community Hospital. contact: Pine Rest Grand Haven Clinic at 616/847-5145

Grand Rapids — Spectrum Health PPD Support Group, meets weekly, contact Nancy Roberts at 616-391-1771 or 616-391-5000

Grand Rapids (Kent County) — Moms Bloom Postpartum Support, visit www.momsbloom.org

St. Clair Shores — Tree of Hope Support Group Call 586-372-6120 or email info@treeofhopefoundation.org.

Sterling Heights — Tree of Hope Support Group Call 586-372-6120 or email info@treeofhopefoundation.org.

Troy — Tree of Hope PPD Support Group Call 586-372-6120 or email info@treeofhopefoundation.org.

MINNESOTA POSTPARTUM DEPRESSION SUPPORT

Minneapolis — PPD Support Group at Abbott NW Mental Health Outpatient Clinic, contact 612-863-4770

Edina — Mindful Monday's for Moms Contact 952-926-BABY http://ammaparentingcenter.com/

St Louis Park — Postpartum Counseling Center: Pregnant & Postpartum Moms Emotional Coping Skills Group:

For more resources, visit the Pregnancy & Postpartum Support Minnesota resource page.

MISSOURI POSTPARTUM DEPRESSION SUPPORT

Maplewood- Support Group held at Amber Sky, contact Gina Rocchio-Gymer at 314-780-349 or at wellnesswithinstl@gmail.com

The Doula Foundation and Ozarks Counseling Center, 1st and 3rd Tuesday of each month
6-8 pm. Located at the Downtown Ward YMCA 417 S. Jefferson Ave.
Springfield, Mo 65806
Please call The Doula Foundation at 417-832-9222 to register. Registration is required.

MONTANA POSTPARTUM DEPRESSION SUPPORT

Bozeman — Deaconess Health Services free PPD support group; meets every Thursday from 6 p.m. to 8 p.m. in the Sapphire Room; contact 406-414-1644

Missoula — PPD Support Group, meets 4th Monday of each month at 10:30am, contact Lara Mattson Radle at 406-370-7747 or email laborandlove@bresnan.net

NEBRASKA POSTPARTUM DEPRESSION SUPPORT

For help in Nebraska, call the Nebraska Dept of Health & Human Services Helpline at 1-800-862-1889

NEVADA POSTPARTUM DEPRESSION SUPPORT

Las Vegas — PPD Support Group at Barbara Greenspun Women's Care Center West. Contact Megan Keith at 702-351-0752

Reno – New Mother's Group. Contact 775-453-4143 for more information or email group@greatbasinwellness.com

NEW HAMPSHIRE POSTPARTUM DEPRESSION SUPPORT

Concord — PPD Support Group. Contact Gerry Mitchell at 603-227-7000 x 4927

Manchester — Postpartum Emotional Support Group at Elliot Hospital's Elliot Childcare Center; contact Alison Palmer with any questions at 663-8927 or palmer1@elliot-hs.org.

Portsmouth – PPD Support Group – Mother-to-Mother Connections – every Tuesday morning from 9-10 a.m. at Families First in Portsmouth, NH. Facilitator: Susan Remillard

NEW JERSEY POSTPARTUM DEPRESSION SUPPORT

http://www.state.nj.us/health/fhs/postpartumdepression

Asbury Park – SPANISH SPEAKING GROUP – Community Affairs & Resource Center, contact Jackie Ramirez at 732-774-3282

Chatham – The Postpartum Place, PPD Circle, contact Laura Winters at 862-200-7218 or visit http://www.postpartumhh.com/support-groups.html

Denville – St. Clare's Behavioral Health, contact 888-626-2111 and ask for moms support group

Dover -- Hope House (Spanish) 19-21 Belmont Avenue, 973-361-5555x 110

Edison – JFK Medical Center, PPD Support Group, contact Donna Weeks at 732-744-5968

Englewood – Englewood Hospital, 50 Engle Street, Teresa Stanley, 201-894-3784,

The Family Success Center, Mommy & Me Support Group, contact Alana Alleyne at 201-568-0817 ext 113

Flemington – Parenting Support Group, Hunterdon Medical Center Education, contact 908-788-6400 #4

Flemington – SPANISH SPEAKING GROUP – Joys of Motherhood, Hunterdon Behavioral Health, contact Florence Francis at 908-788-6401 ext.3107

Flemington- Postpartum Support of Central Jersey. Contact Helen at 908-788-5551 or visit www.Facebook.com/centraljerseypostpartum

Hackensack -- Postpartum Women's Support Group, 547 Main Street, Kim Agresta, 201-784-6718

Hoboken – Hoboken University Medical Center, 201-418-2690

Freehold – New Moms Support Group, CentraState Medical Center, contact 732-308-0570 or www.centrastate.com/healthprograms

Hamilton – Capital Health Medical Center in Hamilton Childbirth & Parent Education Dept., contact 609-303-4140 or www.capitalhealth.org/childbirth

Livingston – Barnabas Health Medical Center, Mommies Moods, contact 973-322-5360

Long Branch – PPD/A Support Group, Monmouth Medical Center, contact Lisa Tremayne at 732-923-5573 or www.barnabashealth.org/mmcPPD

Long Branch – New Moms Support Group, Monmouth Medical Center, contact Theresa Sabella at 732-923-6692

Montclair -- Montclair B.A.B.Y New Moms' Wellness Group, 113 Walnut St., 973-370-0745

Mt. Laurel – TLC for Moms PPD Support Group, contact Virtua Health at 866-380-2229 or www.Virtua.org

Neptune – Meets in Jackson. Contact 732-776-4281 for more information.

New Brunswick – Adjust to the First Year of Motherhood, St. Peters University Hospital, contact Donna Makris at 732-745-8579

New Brunswick – New Moms New Babies Support Group, Robert Wood Johnson University Hospital , contact Betty Pro at 732-253-3871

Newark — PPD Support Group at UMDNJ, (Spanish speaking), contact Sarahjane Rath at 973-972-6216

Paramus — PPD Support Group at Valley Hospital Luckow Pavilion, contact Trudy Heerema at 201-447-8539

Paterson -- New Mothers' Group, St. Joseph's Regional Medical Center – The Giggles Theater, Seton Building – 2nd Floor, 703 Main Street, Audra Burton-Eaterbrook, 973-754-3361

Paterson Public Library, 250 Broadway, The Assembly Room, Martha Amarante, 973-904-0856

Pompton Plains – Chilton Memorial Hospital, 242 West Parkway, Janet Amore, 973-831-5475

Princeton – Postpartum Adjustment Support Group, Princeton Fitness & Wellness Center, contact 609-987-8980

Red Bank – PPD Support Group at Riverview Hospital, contact Karen Edwards at 732-706-5173

Ridgewood – Valley Hospital, Valley Hospital Conference Center, 223 N Van Dien Avenue, Trudy Heerema, 201-447-8539

Rocky Hill — Princeton/Mercer County Postpartum Support Group at Mary Jacobs County Library, contact Joyce Venis at 609-683-1000 (day) or Gail at 732-248-4921 or email joycevenis@yahoo.com

Sewell – Kennedy Health & Wellness Center, Time for Mom Postpartum Wellness, contact 856-582-3098

Spring Lake Heights – Accepting the Unexpected, Natural Beginnings NJ, Resources for Growing Families, contact Samantha Moody at 973-876-5815 or Rebecca McCloskey at 973-876-4283

Somers Point — TLC for Moms PPD Support Group,at Shore Memorial Hospital, contact 609-926-4229

Summit – Overlook Medical Center, Outpatient Behavioral Health, New Mothers Support, contact Patricia Monaghan 908-522-4844

Teaneck — PPD Support Group at Holy Name Hospital, 718 Teaneck Road, contact Ann Anderson at 201-833-3124 or Johanna Gorab, 201-833-3124

Toms River — A Circle of Moms at Community Medical Center, contact Tracy at 732-557-8034

Trenton – Motherhood & More, Mercer Street Friends, contact Elizabeth 609-278-6907

Turnersville – Meridian Counseling Services, Postpartum Moms Support Group, contact 856 -751-0505

Voorhees — Virtua Health, TLC for Moms PPD Support Group, contact 1-866-380-2229

Waldwick -- Women's Wellness Center of Bergen County, 71 Franklin Turnpike, 201-256-3870

NEW MEXICO POSTPARTUM DEPRESSION SUPPORT

Santa Fe — Postpartum Mother's Support Group, meets 11am to noon, contact 505-982-9375

NEW YORK POSTPARTUM DEPRESSION SUPPORT

Circle of Caring PPD Support Groups in Nassau, Suffolk, Westchester Counties, Brooklyn, Manhattan, Staten Island and the Capital Region and other groups forming throughout New York state, contact the Postpartum Resource Center of New York at 631-422-2255 or For more resources in NY, visit the Postpartum Resource Center of New York's resource page here.

Brooklyn — PPD Support Group, contact www.brooklynppdsupport.org or Molly Peryer at 917-549-6012 or email molly@peryer.org

Long Island (Smithtown) — Mother's Circle of Hope PPD Support Group, meets at St. Catherine of Siena Medical Center, contact 631-862-3330

Long Island (West Islip) — Mothers' Circle of Hope – free, 8-week support group for moms experiencing Perinatal Mood and Anxiety Disorders Support Group; Keep Getting Better Group is an ongoing monthly group for moms who have completed another support group. Each meets at Good Samaritan Hospital Medical Center, for more info call 631-376-HOPE or 631-376-4673.

Manhattan — Seleni Institute offers several support groups. Click here for more info.

Richmond County/Staten Island – PPD Support Group at Richmond University Medical Center meets on the third Saturday of every month; call 718-818-2032

Syracuse — Postpartum Depression Support Group at Crouse Hospital in Syracuse, contact Christine Kowaleski, RN at 315-470-7940 or visit http://crouse.org/familysupport/.

Williamsville — PPD Support Group at Millard Filmore Suburban Hospital, meets 2nd Thursdays of each month from 7 to 8pm, contact Nancy Owen at 716-568-3628 or email nowen@kaleidahealth.org

NORTH CAROLINA POSTPARTUM DEPRESSION SUPPORT

Boone – Moms for Moms is free and open to pregnant and new mothers. Every 1st and 3rd Wednesday of each month from 6-7:30 PM at The Children's Council of Watauga County in Boone, NC (225 Birch St # 3, Boone, NC 28607). A brief preregistration is requested before moms first attend group.
Contact email sophierudisill@thechildrenscouncil.org or call The Children's Council (828-262-5424)

Chapel Hill — PPD Support Group hosted by UNC Center for Women's Mood Disorders, Contact 919-966-3115

Cornelius — PPD Support Group, contact Carol Peindl at 704-947-8115

Durham — Duke Postpartum Support program. Contact 919-681-6840

Greensboro- PPD Support Group. Contact 336-832-6848 or 336-832-6848

Greenville — Hopeful Beginnings PPD Support Group at Vidant Medical Center. Contact Kelly Weaver at 252-847-7848 or kelly.weaver@vidanthealth.com

Raleigh — Rex Hospital hosts support group, contact 919-454-6946

Raleigh — weekly PPD support group in Raleigh; contact info@pesnc.org or visit www.pesnc.org

OHIO POSTPARTUM DEPRESSION SUPPORT

Akron/Cleveland: Contact POEM (Perinatal Outreach & Encouragement) Call Leslie & Danielle at 216.282.4569

Columbus: Contact POEM (Perinatal Outreach & Encouragement) Call 614.315.8989 or email Tonya tfulwider@mhafc.org or Amy aburt@mhafc.org

Cincinnati: Contact POEM (Perinatal Outreach & Encouragement) Call Megan at 513.652.3747 or email emlizkadiz@aim.com

Cincinnati – A Lighter Shade of Blue Support Groups, check Facebook page for dates and times or email alightershadeofblue2@yahoo.com.

Chillcothe: Contact POEM (Perinatal Outreach & Encouragement) Call 740.601.9992 or email Jen at jen@poemonline.org or Tandy tandy@poemonline.org

Dayton: Contact POEM (Perinatal Outreach & Encouragement) Call 937.401.6844

Lakewood — Circle of Life Birth and Family Services support group; contact circleoflifebirthservices@gmail.com or call 216-299-8522.

Newark — Contact POEM (Perinatal Outreach & Encouragement)

Contact Christina at poemnewark@gmail.com.

Youngstown: Contact POEM (Perinatal Outreach & Encouragement) Call Leslie, 330.550.2838

OKLAHOMA POSTPARTUM DEPRESSION SUPPORT

Enid — momsTOmoms Support Group. Contact 580-242-4673 for more information.

Midwest City- Moms Support Group Contact Shireen Smith LPC at 405-737-1132 ext 4.

Tulsa — PPD Support Group. For more information visit: http://www.postpartumsupporttulsa.org/#!support-group/c1rd6

OREGON POSTPARTUM DEPRESSION SUPPORT

Eugene & Springfield — WellMama Oregon Support Group info

Portland, Beaverton & Vancouver — Baby Blues Connection PPD Support Groups info

You can also call the WellMama Oregon Warmline at 1-800-896-0410

PENNSYLVANIA POSTPARTUM DEPRESSION SUPPORT

Allentown – Lehigh Valley Health Network Postpartum Support Group: Understanding Emotions after Delivery; call – (610) 402-CARE (2273) for more information on dates/times/location or to register (preferred)

Carlisle – The HOPE Group (Hold On Postpartum Ends); located at The Women's Center at Carlisle Regional Medical Center; call (717) 960-3409 for more information on dates/times

Lancaster – Moms Supporting Moms Group at Community Services building 630 Janet Ave., Lancaster; Call – (717) 397-7461 for more information on dates/times

Lemoyne – Mom's Place PPD Support Group located at 20 Erford Road, Suite 11, Lemoyne; contact (717) 763-2200 for more information on dates/times

Media- Pregnancy and Postpartum Stress Support Group

Philadelphia area — Postpartum Stress Center PPD Support Group info

Philadelphia – Center for Growth

Phoenixville – Postpartum Adjustment Support Group at Phoenixville Hospital Medical Office Building II Third Floor, Conference Center; call (610) 9831415 for more information on dates/times

Pittsburgh – Out of the Blue: free, weekly, drop-in support – Wednesdays 1-3 at Lawrenceville Family Care Connection, 5235 Butler Street, Pittsburgh, PA 15201: Contact Amy Lewis, LCSW amy@socialemotionalchange.com, (412) 532-6622 with any questions or to confirm before first attendance

Pittsburgh – Baby Steps Support Group at St. Clair Hospital Fourth Floor Medical Library; contact (412) 942-5877

West Chester – Postpartum Support Adjustment Group, 790 E Market Street Ste 195, West Chester; contact (610) 931-5547 for more information on dates/times

RHODE ISLAND POSTPARTUM DEPRESSION SUPPORT

Providence — Postpartum Adjustment Group at Women & Infants' Health Education Department, call the warmline at 1-800-711-7011

Providence — Women's Behavioral Medicine

SOUTH CAROLINA POSTPARTUM DEPRESSION SUPPORT

Charleston Area PPD Support Groups: East Cooper Area – East Cooper Medical Center; North Area – Trident Medical Community Center; Downtown – Center for Women; mail: contact@ppdsupport.org or visit http://www.ppdsupport.org/support-group/

Upstate SC — PPD Group of the Upstate. Contact Susan at 864-419-3289

TENNESSEE POSTPARTUM DEPRESSION SUPPORT

Jefferson City (Knoxville area) – Life Outreach Center – Contact Leanne at gizmorgan82@yahoo.com or 615-427-5668.

Nashville – Hope Clinic for Women – Every Wednesday for 6 weeks, starting April 6th, 2016. Contact: Katie Jordan at kjordan@hopeclinicforwomen.org. 615-515-6920

TEXAS POSTPARTUM DEPRESSION SUPPORT

Austin – PPD Support Group at Any Baby Can in Austin. Contact 512-454-3743 or email drkellyboyd@yahoo.com. Spanish capabilities.

Austin – The Circle: Austin Born. 5555 N. Lamar Blvd. c127 Austin. Contact 512-222-5655 or info@austin-born.com or www.counselingfornewmoms.com

Austin – "Mamas for Mamas" Mondays. Contact 512-920-3737 or email info@melissabentley.net

Dallas – Pre/Postpartum Support Group. Contact Karen Erschen at karen@wingsforwellness.org or visit www.wingsforwellness.org

Houston — Center for Postpartum Family Health PPD Support Group. Contact 713-561-3884.

Houston — Mother to Mother support group, sponsored by Texas Children's Hospital. Parking is free. Contact 832-826-5281.

Houston — The Women's Hospital of Texas PPD Support Group. Contact Barbara Crotty at 713-791-7404 or email barbara.crotty@hcahealthcare.com

San Antonio — Methodist Women's Center PPD Support Group. Contact 210-575-0355

San Antonio – Starlight Moms Contact 210-290-3233 or starlightmoms@gmail.com

Tyler — Wings4Moms PPD Support Group. Contact Lindsey Sears at 903-805-2937

http://www.postpartumprogress.com/ppd-support-groups-in-the-u-s-canada - top

UTAH POSTPARTUM DEPRESSION SUPPORT

Salt Lake — Moms and Moods Postpartum Support Group

Sandy — Alta View Hospital PPD Support

Springville – Community Health Clinic Postpartum Support Group *Not Free.

VERMONT POSTPARTUM DEPRESSION SUPPORT

Brattleboro- The Mother's Circle meets at the Winston Prouty Center. For information call 802-258-2414 x213, text 413-522-9451 or email Alison@winstonpouty.org

VIRGINIA POSTPARTUM DEPRESSION SUPPORT

Postpartum Support Virginia Support Groups — for times and locations visit: http://www.postpartumva.org/support-groups/

Manassas — Prince William Medical Center — Hilton Birthing Center. Contact Nancy Sonnenberg, 703-369-8649

Portsmouth — *Military member and dependents.* Portsmouth Naval Medical Center – Contact Kimberly Barnard-Bracey, 757-953-5861

Washington DC — Pregnant and New Moms Group. Contact Lynne McIntyre, 202-545-2061, info@postpartumsupportdc.org

WASHINGTON DC POSTPARTUM DEPRESSION SUPPORT

DC — PPD Support Group, meets Wednesday evenings at Wisconsin Avenue Baptist church, contact Michelle High, info@postpartumdc.org and 202-643-7290

DC — PPD Support Group at Sibley Hospital, meets Wednesdays from noon to 1 on 3rd floor, contact Erin Brindle at 202-537-4773

WASHINGTON POSTPARTUM DEPRESSION SUPPORT

Bremerton — Kitsap Hope Circle at Chiropractic Lifestyle Center. Contact Crystal at 360-990-8901 or visit www.kitsaphopecircle.org. FREE

Federal Way — Balance After Birth. For more info please call Kate (206) 427-4692 or email: kate@yourguidinghands.com. $5-10, pay as you can.

Gig Harbor — Gig Harbor/Port Orchard Hope Circle. Contact Erinn and Marie at kitsaphopecircle@gmail.com or visit www.kitsaphopecircle.org

Kirkland — "This Isn't What I Expected" Support Group. Facilitated by Erin Boone and Tish Rogers. Call EvergreenHealth Posptartum Care Center, 425-899-3602 or EvergreenHealth Healthline, 425-899-100 or email parentbaby@evergreenhealth.org. FREE

Moses Lake — Support Group at Crossroads Resource Center. Contact Christy Youngers at 509-765-4425

Olympia — FREE Thurston County support group at United Churches of Olympia. Facilitators: Stacy Dell, MA LMHC (360)-799-5773, Lisa Iverson, MA LMHCA (360)-790-2273 http://www.lisaiverson.net; Robyn Sowers, MA LMFTA (360)-556-6374 http://robynsowerscounseling.com.

Port Angeles – Circle of Hope. Contact Becca at 755-5213.

Poulsbo — Poulsbo Hope Circle. Contact Crystal at 360-990-8901, email kitsaphopecircle@gmail.com or visit www. kitsaphopecircle.org

Redmond – Conversations About Motherhood for moms with children ages 2 and up. Contact conversationsaboutmotherhood@outlook.com. Suggested $10 contribution.

Seattle- Early Days. Contact Meg at earlydaysWS@gmail.com or visit www.earlydays.org . $10 drop-in fee, pay as you can.

Seattle- Life After Birth

Seattle — Adjusting to Parenthood. Facilitated by Mia Edidin, LICSW. For more info call Mia at 206.659.7773 or Mia.Edidin@perinatalsupport.org and website-http://perinatalsupport.org/item/adjusting-to-parenthood/ $10 drop-in fee, pay as you can.

Tacoma – Balance After Birth at Franciscan Medical Building St. Joseph Medical Center. Contact Franciscan

Family Ed at 253-382-8573 or familyeducation@FHShealth.org or www.chifranciscan.org/familyeducation.

Vancouver – Star Meadow Counseling Support Group. Contact 360-952-3070 or visit www.starmeadowncounseling.com

Perinatal Support of Washington also has a warmline at 888.404.PPMD (7763). Find out more information at www.perinatalsuport.org.

WEST VIRGINIA POSTPARTUM DEPRESSION SUPPORT

There are no support groups that we are aware of at this time. If you know of one, please contact us at resources@postpartumprogress.org so that we can add it.

WISCONSIN POSTPARTUM DEPRESSION SUPPORT

Mequon — Adjusting to Motherhood PPD support group. Contact 262-243-7408.

Oshkosh- YMCA 324 Washington. Childcare available. For more information visit www.mom2momoshkosh.com or email mom2momoshkosh@gmail.com. Phone support available at 920-509-0647

CANADA

Alberta Postpartum Depression Support

Calgary — Families Matter hosts PPD support groups, contact 403-205-5178 for times and locations

British Columbia Postpartum Depression Support

Vancouver — The Pacific Post Partum Support Society offers telephone support, weekly support groups and more, visit www.postpartum.org or call 604-255-7999 for the lower mainland Vancouver area or 1-855-255-7999 for other British Columbia

Manitoba Ontario Postpartum Depression Support

Postpartum Depression of Association of Manitoba Groups

Ontario Postpartum Depression Support

Brantford — The Parachute Program – Transitioning to Parenthood, Call 529-755-9482 or visit The Parachute Program

Burlington— Perinatal Mood Disorder Peer Support Group

Cambridge — Cambridge Memorial Hospital, contact Terry Sousa at 519-621-2330 ext 4312

Cambridge– No Woman Left Behind Support Groups- 2 locations. Your Wellness Team on Queen and Yellowwood Nutrition and Wellness. Contact taniar@golden.net or connect with them on Facebook

Georgetown — Perinatal Mood Disorder Peer Support Group

Kitchener— Support Group with Irene Tiegs at Grand River Hospital, 519-749-4300 ext 226

Milton — Perinatal Mood Disorder Peer Support Group

Mississauga/Brampton/Caledon (Ontario) — Postpartum Support Line, contact 905-459-8439 ext 4

Oakville— Perinatal Mood Disorder Peer Support Group

Ottawa — PPD Support offered by Family Services A La Famille, contact 613-725-3601 ext 117 or email intake@familyservicesottawa.org

Toronto — East Toronto Postpartum Adjustment Program, contact 416-469-7608

Windsor/Essex County- Safe Place Postpartum Support

Windsor- Mommy Matters Group. Call 519-255-9940 x135

Saskatchewan Postpartum Depression Support

Regina— Postpartum Support Group at the YMCA of Regina, contact Sally Elliott at 306-757-9622 x 242

Saskatoon— PPD Support Group, contact 306-655-6777

Postpartum Depression Support Groups in the U.S. & Canada

Postpartum Depression Support Groups Around the U.S. &

Canada

ONLINE SUPPORT

Academy of Integrative Health & Medicine:

http://www.AIHM.org
Applying integrative and holistic medicine principles to health."

Center for Complementary and Alternative Medicine:

http://www.nccam.nih.gov
"Expanding horizons of healthcare. By National Institutes of Health."

Center for Postpartum Health:

http://www.postpartumhealth.com
"Where mothers are mothered." Emphasizes assessment and prevention. .

Clearsky:

http://www.clearsky-inc.com
"Finding and keeping joy." Dr. Shoshana Bennett's perinatal depression website.

DBSA: Depression and Bipolar Support Alliance:

http://www.dbsalliance.org
"Improving the lives of people living with mood disorders."

Mothersrisk.org:

http://www.motherrisk.org
Provides links and a search tool for a number of pregnancy-related topics."

NAMI: National Alliance on Mental Illness:

http://www.nami.org
Dedicated to the eradication of mental illness and improvement of quality of life for those affected.

NASPOG: North American Society for Psychosocial Obstetrics and Gynecology:

http://www.naspog.org
Purpose is "to foster scholarly scientific and clinical study of the bio psychosocial aspects of obstetric and gynecologic medicine."

For Spanish-speaking mothers:

Apoyo de PSI Para Las Familias Hispano Parlantes 1-800-944-4772

#1 Llame al numero de telefono gratuito para obtener recursos,

apoyo e informaciou gratuita. Dejenos un mensaje y un voluntario

le devolvera la llamada.

Nueva Vida Posparto Grupo. You will need to send a private

message asking to join the private Facebook group.

Postpartum Resource Ce Postpartum Resource Center of New York:

http://www.postpartumny.org
One of the first organizations to provide state-specific and general information and support to women with PPMDs.

Ruth Rhoden Craven Foundation:

http://www.ppdsupport.org
Online support named after Ruth Craven who died when her son was two and a half months old. The foundation's goal is to provide information and support . . . and to serve as a resource to those in the medical community.

Solace for Mothers: Healing after Traumatic Childbirth:

http://www.solaceformothers.org
Online community with resources for those dealing with recovery from challenging or traumatic childbirth experience. Also has a warmline: 877-SOLACE..

United States Support Groups

Nationwide: Postpartum Support International, Postpartum Progress Inc.

ALABAMA POSTPARTUM DEPRESSION SUPPORT

There are no support groups that we are aware of at this time. If you know of one, please contact us at resources@postpartumprogress.org so that we can add it.

ALASKA POSTPARTUM DEPRESSION SUPPORT

Anchorage — Monday Mama's Support group. Postpartum Support Alaska meets at the Maternity Education Center at the Children's Hospital at Providence. Contact the Family Support Counseling Clinic at 907-212-4940 or Joclyn Reilly, Family Support Services counselor.

Fairbanks – Alaska Family Health & Birth Center Support Group. Contact 907-456-3719 to register

ARIZONA POSTPARTUM DEPRESSION SUPPORT

Arizona Postpartum Wellness Coalition, Tucson Postpartum
Depression Coalition

Flagstaff — Postpartum Adjustment Support Group at North
County Healthcare. Contact 928-707-0748 to register

Gilbert – Pregnancy and Postpartum Support Group at Dignity
Health. Wednesdays from 1 to 2:30 p.m. (Support groups do not
meet week of July 4th, Thanksgiving, Christmas and New Year's)
Free. Moms may bring a support person with them. Infants and
toddlers are welcome. Rome Towers, 1760 E Pecos Rd., #235
Gilbert, AZ 85295

Glendale — New Moms Postpartum Support Group meets at
Banner Thunderbird Medical Center. Contact 602-865-5908

Mesa — Pregnancy and Postpartum Adjustment Support
Group meets Tuesdays from 10-11:30 at Banner Desert Medical
Center; contact 480-412-5292

Phoenix — Mother to Mother support group at St. Joseph's
Hospital, Contact 1-877-602-4111

Tucson — Pregnancy and Postpartum Adjustment Support Group
at Northwest Medical Center. Contact Alison at 520-877-4149

Tucson — Postpartum Depression Support Group at St. Joseph's Hospital. Contact Carole at 520-873-6858

You can also call the Arizona Postpartum Warmline at 1-888-434-MOMS

ARKANSAS POSTPARTUM DEPRESSION SUPPORT

There are no support groups that we are aware of at this time. If you know of one, please contact resources@postpartumprogress.org.

CALIFORNIA POSTPARTUM DEPRESSION SUPPORT

CaPSI Warmline 1-855-227-7462, California Maternal Mental Health Collaborative;

Auburn – Insights Counseling Group. 8207 Sierra College Blvd. Contact (530) 887-1300 or Colleen@insightscounselinggroup.org

Berkeley — North Berkeley Postpartum Stress Support Group. Contact Lee Safran at 510-496-6096

Beverly Hills — What about Mommy? A postpartum Group for Mothers, contact (310) 929-0638

Campbell – Adjusting to Motherhood Emotional Support Group at Tiny Tots. Contact Cheryl Hart at 408-475-4408 or Cheryl@supportingmamas.org

Claremont — Postpartum support group. Email drkaeni@gmail.com or call 909-451-9951.

Clearlake — Mother-Wise. Contact Jaclyn at 707-349-1210 or visit our Facebook page for more event information https://www.facebook.com/MotherWiseLakeCounty

Fresno — Babies R Us. Facilitators: Stephanie Chandler, PM & Susan Kordell, RN. Contact 559-244-4580

Fresno — First 5 Lighthouse for Children 2405 Tulare St. Fresno, 93721. Facilitator: Alejandra Addo-Boateng, MFTI, 559-244-4580

La Jolla — at Scripps Memorial Hospital, call 1-800-SCRIPPS

La Mesa — at Sharp Grossmont Hospital, contact 619-740-4906

Lafayette – Postpartum Emotional Recovery Circle at Mt. Diablo Perinatal Psychotherapy Associates. Contact Meri Levy, MFT at 925-385-8848

Lakeport — Mother-Wise. Contact Jaclyn at 707-349-1210 or visit our Facebook page for more event

information https://www.facebook.com/MotherWiseLakeCounty

Long Beach — Transitioning Into Motherhood support services at Long Beach Memorial.

Visit http://transitionsinmotherhood.com/events/

Los Angeles — LA County Perinatal Mental Health Task Force,

Los Gatos — El Camino Hospital Los Gatos Pregnancy & Postpartum Resiliency Circle; meets during the year in 6-week series; call for dates and times here 650-962-5745.

Madera — Fridays: 9-1030am, Family Resource Center, 525 E. Yosemite Ave. Madera, 93638. Facilitator: Roccio Arevalo, MFTI, bi-lingual English/Spanish, 559-675-4004

Monterey— Postpartum Support Groups. Contact 831-783-5933, email hello@parentingconnectionmc.org. Visit www.parentingconnectionmc.org

Mariposa —The Hub, 5078 Billion St. Mariposa. Facilitator: Jenny Morgan, 559-240-4370

Mission Viejo — Postpartum Adjustment Support Group at Mission Viejo Hospital. Contact Sue Harrison at 949-365-3818

Newport Beach — at Hoag Hospital. Contact Laura Navarro Pickens, LCSW for more information at (562) 882-7901

Oceanside — "Babies in Bloom". Contact Holly Herring, at 760-814-1421

Orange — at St. Joseph Hospital. Contact 714-771-8000 ext. 17891

Pacific Grove — Postpartum Wellness Support Group at Parent's Place. Contact Meg Grundy at 831-601-7021 or email meggrundy@yahoo.com

Pasadena – Motherhood Journey Therapy Groups for new and expectant mothers at the Institute for Girls' Development. Sonia Nikore, LMFT, 84145 at Institute for Girls Development at 626-585-8075 ext. 102

Roseville — PPD Support Group. Contact Kelly McGinnis at shineonsupport@outlook.com or 916-770-9394

San Diego — Postpartum Health Alliance of San Diego; at Sharp Mary Birch Hospital. Contact 858-939-4141

San Francisco — Newborn Connections Postpartum Depression Support Group at California Pacific Medical Center, contact 415-600-2229

San Francisco — 6-week "Afterglow" PPD support group, held several times throughout the year, as part of UCSF Great Expectations Pregnancy program, for more info: http://www.whrc.ucsf.edu/whrc/gex/afterglow.html

San Francisco — Postpartum Support Groups led by Robyn Alagona

San Jose — Supporting Mamas (San Jose area) ; "Adjusting to Motherhood Emotional Support Group at Tiny Tots. Contact Cheryl Hart at 408-475-4408 or Cheryl@supportingmamas.org

San Luis Obispo — Alpha Parenting PPD Support Line, 1-805-541-3367

San Luis Obispo — From a Pea to a Pumpkin prenatal support group. Tuesdays 3:15 – 4:30pm. Contact: (805)884-9794 or angela@angelawurtzelmft.com

Santa Barbara — From a Pea to a Pumpkin prenatal support group. Mondays 1:00 – 2:15pm. Contact: (805)884-9794 or angela@angelawurtzelmft.com

Serra Mesa — at Sharp Mary Birch Hospital. Contact 858-939-4141

Sherman Oaks – Motherhood Journey Postpartum Support Group at BINI Birth. Contact Robin Starkey Harpster, MA

MFT rharpster@instituteforgirlsdevelopment.com 626-585-8075 ext. 109

Sherman Oaks – Postpartum Passages Contact Diana Barnes (818) 887-1312

COLORADO POSTPARTUM DEPRESSION SUPPORT

Boulder — Postpartum Transitions Group at the Postpartum Wellness Center. For more information and to register call 303-335-9473 or email rosie@pwcboulder.com.

Denver — PPD Support Group at Women's Therapy Center Cherry Creek. Contact Avery Neal at 866-995-7910

Healthy Expectations at Children's Hospital of Colorado

Denver – PPD Support at the Catalyst Center. For more information click here

Denver – Afterglow: Postpartum Therapy Group for Struggling Moms or Dads

Littleton — Hope 4 Moms. Contact Mary Anderson Schroeter at 303-883-7271 or mary.schroeter@comcast.net. www.IntergrativePathwaysCounseling.com https://www.facebook.com/h4moms/

CONNECTICUT POSTPARTUM DEPRESSION SUPPORT

Torrington – Charlotte Hungerford Hospital New Mother's Wellness Group, contact Amy Rodriguez at (860) 496-6359

West Hartford – Adjustment to Baby Challenges. Contact Annie Keating-Scherer at (860)212-7066 or Sharon Thomason at (860)331-1750

Connecticut Alliance for Perinatal Mental Health

DELAWARE POSTPARTUM DEPRESSION SUPPORT

Newark, Wilmington & Dover — MOMs HEAL: Perinatal Mood Disorder Support Groups. Contact 302-733-6662 or email cwew@christianacare.org. http://www.christianacare.org/momsheal

FLORIDA POSTPARTUM DEPRESSION SUPPORT

Gainesville — Postpartum Adjustment Support Group

Jacksonville — Baptist Health PPD Support Group, to find out more and register, click here

Tampa – Coping With Motherhood PPD support group and Circle of Hope Group at St. Joseph's Women's Hospital. Contact Kristina Davis at 813-872-3925.

Postpartum Society of Florida

GEORGIA POSTPARTUM DEPRESSION SUPPORT

Atlanta — Atlanta Postpartum Support Group, www.meetup.com/PPDAtlanta, meets monthly, contact Amber Koter at atlantamom930@gmail.com or call 914-261-8182

Carrollton – "Mommy's Day Out" Support Group. Contact Jwyanda Norman at 678-739-740 or email her at jwyanda@cloud.com

Dunwoody — PPD Support Group, contact cassieowenslpc@gmail.com or call 404-448-1733

Marietta — Emerge Into Light PPD support group.

Project Healthy Moms,

You can also call the GA Project Healthy Moms Warmline for support at 1-800-933-9896 ext 234

HAWAII POSTPARTUM DEPRESSION SUPPORT

Oahu — PPD Support Group. Contact Diane at 808-392-7985

IDAHO POSTPARTUM DEPRESSION SUPPORT

Boise/Nampa — at St. Alphonsus Regional Medical Center, contact 208-367-7380

Ketchum — at the Center for Community Health. Contact 208-727-8733

Moscow — at Gritman Medical Center, contact 208-883-6385

PPD Support HI

ILLINOIS POSTPARTUM DEPRESSION SUPPORT

Postpartum Depression Alliance of Illinois, Melanie's Battle

Chicago — Postpartum Depression Program at Healthcare Alternative Systems; Free services in English and Spanish. Contact 773-292-4242

Chicago — Transitions to Motherhood program at Northwestern Memorial's Prentice Women's Hospital; Register by calling 312-926-8400

Elk Grove – Door of Hope PPD support group at Alexian Brothers Medical Center; contact Lita Simanis at 847-981-3644 or lita.simanis@alexian.net

Elk Grove – La Maternidad y Yo: Spanish-language support group for new and expectant moms at Alexian Brothers Medical Center; contact Natasha Varela at 847 755 8447 or Natasha.varela@alexian.net

Evanston — Beyond the Baby Blues PPD Support Group. Contact 847-864-7957; www.beyondthebabyblues.org

Fathers' Support Groups: Hoffman Estates — MVP Men vs. Postpartum – Support group for fathers who have loved ones experiencing PPD; Contact Lita Simanis at 847-755-3220

Fathers' Support Groups –
http://www.postpartumdads.org

Glenview — Pregnancy and Postpartum Support Group at Courage to Connect. Contact kelly@couragetoconnecttherapy.com or 847-730-3042

Hinsdale — PPD Support Group; call 630-856-4390.

Hoffman Estates — PPD support group. Contact Lita Simanis at 847-755-3220

Northbrook – New Mom Support Group meets 2nd Wednesday of the month.

Oak Lawn — meets at Advocate Christ Conference Center. Contact 708-684-1333

Oak Park — at Parenthesis Parent Child Center, contact Mary Strizak at 708-848-2227 or email mstrizak@parenthesis-info.org

Springfield—Postpartum Depression Support Group at HSHS St. John's Hospital—"New Moms Dealing with Feelings." Contact the Parent Help Line(a toll-free confidential phone line) at 1-888-727-5889 or 1-217-544-5808 or email elizabeth.krah@hshs.org.

Winfield — at Central DuPage Hospital, meets Wednesdays from 11-12:30pm and Thursdays from 6:30-8pm; contact 630-933-1964

** For more Illinois support group information and resources, visit PPDIL

INDIANA POSTPARTUM DEPRESSION SUPPORT

Indiana Perinatal Network

Ft. Wayne — Lutheran Hospital support group, contact Michelle Dearmond, RN,BS, IBCLC at 260-435

7069 or mdearmond2@lutheran-hospital.com

Indianapolis — Indiana University Health, Contact Birdie Meyer at 317-962-8191 bmeyer2@iuhealth.org,

Indianapolis — Community Health Support group; Contact Marcia Boring MSW, LCSW, at 317-621-7828 or mboring@community.com

Indianapolis — Hendricks Regional Health support group; contact Brittany Waggoner, RN, BSN, CNS at 317-718-4018 or bswaggo@hendricks.org

Lafayette — Kathryn Weil Center support group; Contact 765-449-5133

South Bend — Mother Matters support group at South Bend Memorial Hospital, contact 574-647-3243 (or pager 574-236-7811, 8am-10pm)

South Bend — Peer support group for new moms at Good Shepherd Lutheran Church; Contact Linda Meeks at 574 272-3446

IOWA POSTPARTUM DEPRESSION SUPPORT

Cedar Rapids — Murray, Wilson & Rose. Contact 319-213-6010

Des Moines – Pine Rest Des Moines Support Group, contact 515-331-0303

KANSAS POSTPARTUM DEPRESSION SUPPORT

Pregnancy & Postpartum Resource Center

Lawrence — at Lawrence Memorial Hospital (newborns welcome); Contact 785-505-3081 for more info

Overland Park —Contact the Postpartum Resource Center of Kansas at 913-677-1300

Shawnee Mission — Shawnee Mission Medical Center Postpartum Emotional Support Group

South Jackson County — Contact the Postpartum Resource Center of Kansas at 913-677-1300

Topeka – Sacred Circle of Northeast Kansas

KENTUCKY POSTPARTUM DEPRESSION SUPPORT

Postpartum Support Kentuckiana

Lexington – The Postpartum Adjustment Center Contact 859-327-6459

For support you can also call the Postpartum Support Kentuckiana warmline at 502-541-1818

LOUISIANA POSTPARTUM DEPRESSION SUPPORT

Zachary – Lane Medical Center PPD Support Group, call 225-658-4587

MAINE POSTPARTUM DEPRESSION SUPPORT

Brunswick — PPD Support Group at Mid Coast Hospital, contact 207-373-6500 * Starting back up January 2016

MARYLAND POSTPARTUM DEPRESSION SUPPORT

Healthy New Moms; Postpartum Support Maryland

Annapolis — at Anne Arundel Medical Center, Contact Ali Tiedke at 443-481-6124 or email atiedke@aahs.org

Baltimore — Postpartum Support Group at Sinai Hospital, contact Sara Daly, LCSW-C at 410-601-7832 or skdaly@lifebridgehealth.org

Elkton — Moms Matter Postpartum Support Group –Contact Beth Chipriano 410-620-3773 or bchipriano@uhcc.com.

Silver Spring — PPD support group at Holy Cross Resource Center, free & no registration required, meets 1st and 3rd Sundays from 6-7:30pm; contact: MDpostpartum@gmail.com

MASSACHUSETTS POSTPARTUM DEPRESSION SUPPORT

North Shore Postpartum Depression Task Force, MotherWoman, South Shore Postpartum Support Network

Acton – Emotional Wellbeing After Baby group at First Connections, 179 Great Road, Suite 104; Contact Laurie Ganberg at 978-287-0221, lganberg@jri.org. http://www.firstconnections.org/

Brookline – Support Group $25/session, Contact Rachel Kalvert, LICSW at 617-487-1521

Greenfield – Franklin County Postpartum Support Group at the Community Action Family Center, 90 Federal Street; Contact Sandy Clark at 413-475-1566, http://www.communityaction.us/

Holyoke – MotherWoman Postpartum Support at Midwifery Care of Holyoke, 230 Maple Street, (413) 534 – 2700, http://www.motherwoman.org/

North Reading – Postpartum Adjustment Support Groups at Stork Ready, 325 Mani Street; Contact Leslie McKeough at 781-507-2025, lamckeough@gmail.com, http://www.corevalu.com/

Newton – "Balance With Baby" Postpartum Support Group at The Freedman Center at William James College, One Wells Ave; Contact Chardae Golding at 617-332-3666 x 1123, Email: freedmancenter@williamjames.edu, http://www.williamjames.edu/community/freedman-center/index.cfm

Newton – Free Support Groups: http://www.williamjames.edu/community/freedman-center/new-moms.cfm

Plymouth – Depression After Delivery at Jordan Hospital, 275 Sandwich St., Meditation Room; Contact Gerri Piatelli at 781-837-4242, http://www.bidplymouth.org

Waltham – "This Isn't What I Expected" PPD Support Group at JF&CS, 1430 Main Street; Contact Debbie Whitehill at 781-647-5327 x1925, dwhitehill@jfcsboston.org, http://www.jfcsboston.org/

Watertown – Strong Roots PPD Support Groups, find information here.

MICHIGAN POSTPARTUM DEPRESSION SUPPORT

Tree of Hope Foundation, Moms Bloom

Bay City — Depression After Delivery Support Group, contact Sherry LaMere or Kelli Wilkinson at 989-895-2240

Clawson — Nature's Playhouse Traumatic Birth Support group, No registration necessary. Children are welcome. www.naturesplayhouse.com

Flint — PPD Support Group at Hurley Medical Center, no contact info available

Grand Haven — PPD Support Group at North Ottawa Community Hospital. contact: Pine Rest Grand Haven Clinic at 616/847-5145

Grand Rapids — Spectrum Health PPD Support Group, meets weekly, contact Nancy Roberts at 616-391-1771 or 616-391-5000

Grand Rapids (Kent County) — Moms Bloom Postpartum Support, visit www.momsbloom.org

St. Clair Shores — Tree of Hope Support Group Call 586-372-6120 or email info@treeofhopefoundation.org.

Sterling Heights — Tree of Hope Support Group Call 586-372-6120 or email info@treeofhopefoundation.org.

Troy — Tree of Hope PPD Support Group Call 586-372-6120 or email info@treeofhopefoundation.org.

MINNESOTA POSTPARTUM DEPRESSION SUPPORT

Jenny's Light, Pregnancy & Postpartum Support Minnesota

Minneapolis — PPD Support Group at Abbott NW Mental Health Outpatient Clinic, contact 612-863-4770

Edina — Mindful Monday's for Moms Contact 952-926-BABY

http://ammaparentingcenter.com/

For more resources, visit the Pregnancy & Postpartum Support Minnesota resource page.

MISSOURI POSTPARTUM DEPRESSION SUPPORT

Maplewood- Support Group held at Amber Sky, contact Gina Rocchio-Gymer at 314-780-349 or at wellnesswithinstl@gmail.com

MONTANA POSTPARTUM DEPRESSION SUPPORT

Bozeman — Deaconess Health Services free PPD support group; meets every Thursday from 6 p.m. to 8 p.m. in the Sapphire Room; contact 406-414-1644

Missoula — PPD Support Group, meets 4th Monday of each month at 10:30am, contact Lara Mattson Radle at 406-370-7747 or email laborandlove@bresnan.net

NEBRASKA POSTPARTUM DEPRESSION SUPPORT

For help in Nebraska, call the Nebraska Dept of Health & Human Services Helpline at 1-800-862-1889

NEVADA POSTPARTUM DEPRESSION SUPPORT

Las Vegas — Beyond Birth Postpartum Support Group, meets Wednesdays at 1pm at Family to Family at 4412 S. Maryland Parkway, contact 631-7098

Las Vegas — PPD Support Group at Barbara Greenspun Women's Care Center West, meets Mondays from 10-11am, contact Megan Keith at 702/351-0752 or keithfazolis@earthlink.net

Las Vegas — PPD Support Group at the OBGYN Specialists, meets 1st and 3rd Wednesday of each month from 7-8pm, contact Vanessa Delorenzis at 702/577-8039 or delorenzis2002@hotmail.com

Las Vegas — PPD Support Group at Pinkpeas Pregnancy and Parenting Care Center, meets every other Thursday from 2-3pm, contact Vanessa Delorenzis at 702/577-8039 or delorenzis2002@hotmail.com

NEW HAMPSHIRE POSTPARTUM DEPRESSION SUPPORT

Concord — PPD Support Group. Contact Gerry Mitchell at 603-227-7000 x 4927

Manchester — Postpartum Emotional Support Group at Elliot Hospital's Elliot Childcare Center; contact Alison Palmer with any questions at 663-8927 or palmer1@elliot-hs.org.

Portsmouth – PPD Support Group – Mother-to-Mother Connections – every Tuesday morning from 9-10 a.m. at Families First in Portsmouth, NH. Facilitator: Susan Remillard

NEW JERSEY POSTPARTUM DEPRESSION SUPPORT

Southern New Jersey Perinatal Cooperative, Partnership for Maternal & Child Health of Northern New Jersey

Asbury Park – SPANISH SPEAKING GROUP – Community Affairs & Resource Center, contact Jackie Ramirez at 732-774-3282

Chatham – The Postpartum Place, PPD Circle, contact Laura Winters at 862-200-7218 or visit http://www.postpartumhh.com/support-groups.html

Denville – St. Clare's Behavioral Health, contact 888-626-2111 and ask for moms support group

Edison – JFK Medical Center, PPD Support Group, contact Donna Weeks at 732-744-5968

Englewood – The Family Success Center, Mommy & Me Support Group, contact Alana Alleyne at 201-568-0817 ext 113

Flemington – Parenting Support Group, Hunterdon Medical Center Education, contact 908-788-6400 #4

Flemington – SPANISH SPEAKING GROUP – Joys of Motherhood, Hunterdon Behavioral Health, contact Florence Francis at 908-788-6401 ext.3107

Hoboken – Hoboken University Medical Center, 201-418-2690

Freehold – New Moms Support Group, CentraState Medical Center, contact 732-308-0570 or www.centrastate.com/healthprograms

Hamilton – Capital Health Medical Center in Hamilton Childbirth & Parent Education Dept., contact 609-303-4140 or www.capitalhealth.org/childbirth

Livingston – Barnabas Health Medical Center, Mommies Moods, contact 973-322-5360

Long Branch – PPD/A Support Group, Monmouth Medical Center, contact Lisa Tremayne at 732-923-5573 or www.barnabashealth.org/mmcPPD

Long Branch – New Moms Support Group, Monmouth Medical Center, contact Theresa Sabella at 732-923-6692

Mt. Laurel – TLC for Moms PPD Support Group, contact Virtua Health at 866-380-2229 or www.Virtua.org

Neptune – Meets in Jackson. Contact 732-776-4281 for more information.

New Brunswick – Adjust to the First Year of Motherhood, St. Peters University Hospital, contact Donna Makris at 732-745-8579

New Brunswick – New Moms, New Babies Support Group, Robert Wood Johnson University Hospital , contact Betty Pro at 732-253-3871

Newark — PPD Support Group at UMDNJ, (Spanish speaking), contact Sarahjane Rath at 973-972-6216

Paramus — PPD Support Group at Valley Hospital Luckow Pavilion, contact Trudy Heerema at 201-447-8539

Princeton – Postpartum Adjustment Support Group, Princeton Fitness & Wellness Center, contact 609-987-8980

Red Bank – PPD Support Group at Riverview Hospital, contact Karen Edwards at 732-706-5173

Rocky Hill — Princeton/Mercer County Postpartum Support Group at Mary Jacobs County Library, contact Joyce Venis at 609-683-1000 (day) or Gail at 732-248-4921 or email joycevenis@yahoo.com

Sewell – Kennedy Health & Wellness Center, Time for Mom Postpartum Wellness, contact 856-582-3098

Spring Lake Heights – Accepting the Unexpected, Natural Beginnings NJ, Resources for Growing Families, contact Samantha Moody at 973-876-5815 or Rebecca McCloskey at 973-876-4283

Somers Point — TLC for Moms PPD Support Group,at Shore Memorial Hospital, contact 609-926-4229

Summit – Overlook Medical Center, Outpatient Behavioral Health, New Mothers Support, contact Patricia Monaghan 908-522-4844

Teaneck — PPD Support Group at Holy Name Hospital, contact Ann Anderson at 201-833-3124

Toms River — A Circle of Moms at Community Medical Center, contact Tracy at 732-557-8034

Trenton – Motherhood & More, Mercer Street Friends, contact Elizabeth 609-278-6907

Turnersville – Meridian Counseling Services, Postpartum Moms Support Group, contact 856 -751-0505

Voorhees — Virtua Health, TLC for Moms PPD Support Group, contact 1-866-380-2229

NEW MEXICO POSTPARTUM DEPRESSION SUPPORT

Santa Fe — Postpartum Mother's Support Group, meets 11am to noon, contact 505-982-9375

NEW YORK POSTPARTUM DEPRESSION SUPPORT

The Postpartum Resource Center of New York, Shades of Light (Capital Region), Perinatal Network of New York

Circle of Caring PPD Support Groups in Nassau, Suffolk, Westchester Counties, Brooklyn, Manhattan, Staten Island and the Capital Region and other groups forming throughout New York state, contact the Postpartum Resource Center of New York at 631-422-2255 or For more resources in NY, visit the Postpartum Resource Center of New York's resource page here.

Brooklyn — PPD Support Group, contact www.brooklynppdsupport.org or Molly Peryer at 917-549-6012 or email molly@peryer.org

Long Island (Smithtown) — Mother's Circle of Hope PPD Support Group, meets at St. Catherine of Siena Medical Center, contact 631-862-3330

Long Island (West Islip) — Mothers' Circle of Hope – free, 8-week support group for moms experiencing Perinatal Mood and Anxiety Disorders Support Group; Keep Getting Better Group is an ongoing monthly group for moms who have completed another support group. Each meets at Good Samaritan Hospital Medical Center, for more info call 631-376-HOPE or 631-376-4673.

Manhattan — Seleni Institute offers several support groups. Click here for more info.

Richmond County/Staten Island – PPD Support Group at Richmond University Medical Center meets on the third Saturday of every month; call 718-818-2032

Syracuse — Postpartum Depression Support Group at Crouse Hospital in Syracuse, contact Christine Kowaleski, RN at 315-470-7940 or visit http://crouse.org/familysupport/.

Williamsville — PPD Support Group at Millard Filmore Suburban Hospital, meets 2nd Thursdays of each month from 7 to 8pm, contact Nancy Owen at 716-568-3628 or email nowen@kaleidahealth.org

NORTH CAROLINA POSTPARTUM DEPRESSION SUPPORT

: Postpartum Education & Support

Chapel Hill — PPD Support Group hosted by UNC Center for Women's Mood Disorders, Contact 919-966-3115

Cornelius — PPD Support Group, contact Carol Peindl at 704-947-8115

Durham — Duke Postpartum Support program. Contact 919-681-6840

Greenville — Hopeful Beginnings PPD Support Group at Vidant Medical Center. Contact Kelly Weaver at 252-847-7848 or kelly.weaver@vidanthealth.com

Raleigh — Rex Hospital hosts support group, contact 919-454-6946

Raleigh — weekly PPD support group in Raleigh; contact info@pesnc.org or visit www.pesnc.org

NORTH DAKOTA POSTPARTUM DEPRESSION SUPPORT

Pregnancy & Postpartum Support North Dakota

OHIO POSTPARTUM DEPRESSION SUPPORT

Perinatal Outreach & Encouragement for Moms (POEM)

Akron/Cleveland: Contact POEM (Perinatal Outreach & Encouragement) Call Leslie & Danielle at 216.282.4569

Columbus: Contact POEM (Perinatal Outreach & Encouragement) Call 614.315.8989 or email Tonya tfulwider@mhafc.org or Amy aburt@mhafc.org

Cincinnati: Contact POEM (Perinatal Outreach & Encouragement) Call Megan at 513.652.3747 or email emlizkadiz@aim.com

Cincinnati – A Lighter Shade of Blue Support Groups, check Facebook page for dates and times or email alightershadeofblue2@yahoo.com.

Cleveland — PPD Support Group, for more info call 216-373-0302.

Chillcothe: Contact POEM (Perinatal Outreach & Encouragement) Call 740.601.9992 or email Jen at jen@poemonline.org or Tandy tandy@poemonline.org

Dayton: Contact POEM (Perinatal Outreach & Encouragement) Call 937.401.6844

Lakewood — Circle of Life Birth and Family Services support group; contact circleoflifebirthservices@gmail.com or call 216-299-8522.

Newark — Moms Offering Mothers Support, PPD & anxiety support group, contact momsforlife43055@gmail.com.

Youngstown: Contact POEM (Perinatal Outreach & Encouragement) Call Leslie, 330.550.2838

OKLAHOMA POSTPARTUM DEPRESSION SUPPORT

Enid — momsTOmoms Support Group. Contact 580-242-4673 for more information.

Midwest City- Moms Support Group Contact Shireen Smith LPC at 405-737-1132 ext 4.

Tulsa — PPD Support Group. For more information visit: http://www.postpartumsupporttulsa.org/#!support-group/c1rd6

OREGON POSTPARTUM DEPRESSION SUPPORT

Eugene & Springfield — WellMama Oregon Support Group info

Portland, Beaverton & Vancouver — Baby Blues Connection PPD Support Groups info

You can also call the WellMama Oregon Warmline at 1-800-896-0410

PENNSYLVANIA POSTPARTUM DEPRESSION SUPPORT

Allentown – Lehigh Valley Health Network Postpartum Support Group: Understanding Emotions after Delivery; call – (610) 402-CARE (2273) for more information on dates/times/location or to register (preferred)

Carlisle – The HOPE Group (Hold On Postpartum Ends); located at – The Women's Center at Carlisle Regional Medical Center; call – (717) 960-3409 for more information on dates/times

Ephrata – Mother to Mother PPD peer support group; located at – Ephrata Public Library Conference Room; contact – MTMLancaster@gmail.com for more information on dates/times

Lancaster – Moms Supporting Moms Group; located at – Community Services building 630 Janet Ave., Lancaster; call – (717) 397-7461 for more information on dates/times

Lemoyne – Mom's Place PPD Support Group; located at – 20 Erford Road, Suite 11, Lemoyne; call – (717) 763-2200 for more information on dates/times

Philadelphia area — Postpartum Stress Center PPD Support Group info

Philadelphia – Center for Growth

Phoenixville – Postpartum Adjustment Support Group; location – Phoenixville Hospital Medical Office Building II Third Floor, Conference Center; call – (610) 9831415 for more information on dates/times

Pittsburgh – Out of the Blue Support Group; located at – Shining Light Prenatal Education 3701 Butler St. Pittsburgh; call – Amy Lewis amy@socialemotionalchange.com, (412) 532-6622 before first attendance to confirm dates/times

Pittsburgh – <u>Baby</u> Steps Support Group; located at – St. Clair Hospital Fourth Floor Medical Library; call – (412) 942-5877

West Chester – Postpartum Support Adjustment Group; located at – 790 E Market Street Ste 195, West Chester; call – (610) 931-5547 for more information on dates/times

RHODE ISLAND POSTPARTUM DEPRESSION SUPPORT

Providence — Postpartum Adjustment Group at Women & Infants' Health Education Department, call the warmline at 1-800-711-7011

SOUTH CAROLINA POSTPARTUM DEPRESSION SUPPORT

Charleston Area PPD Support Groups: East Cooper Area – East Cooper Medical Center; North Area – Trident Medical Community Center; Downtown – Center for Women; mail: contact@ppdsupport.org or visit http://www.ppdsupport.org/support-group/

Upstate SC — PPD Group of the Upstate. Contact Susan at 864-419-3289

<u>Ruth Rhoden Craven Foundation</u>,

for Spanish speakers: PASOs; Postpartum Support Charleston

TENNESSEE POSTPARTUM DEPRESSION SUPPORT

Nashville – Hope Clinic for Women – Every Wednesday for 6 weeks, starting April 6th, 2016. Contact: Katie Jordan at kjordan@hopeclinicforwomen.org. 615-515-6920

There are no more support groups that we are aware of at this time. If you know of one, please contact us at resources@postpartumprogress.org so that we can add it.

TEXAS POSTPARTUM DEPRESSION SUPPORT

Austin – PPD Support Group at Any Baby Can in Austin. Contact 512-454-3743 or email drkellyboyd@yahoo.com. Spanish capabilities.

Pregnancy & Postpartum Health Alliance of Texas

Austin – The Circle: Austin Born. 5555 N. Lamar Blvd. c127 Austin. Contact 512-222-5655 or info@austin-born.com or www.counselingfornewmoms.com

Austin – "Mamas for Mamas" Mondays. Contact 512-920-3737 or email info@melissabentley.net

Dallas – Pre/Postpartum Support Group. Contact Karen Erschen at karen@wingsforwellness.org or visit www.wingsforwellness.org

Houston — Center for Postpartum Family Health PPD Support Group. Contact 713-561-3884.

Houston — Mother to Mother support group, sponsored by Texas Children's Hospital. Parking is free. Contact 832-826-5281.

Houston — The Women's Hospital of Texas PPD Support Group. Contact Barbara Crotty at 713-791-7404 or email barbara.crotty@hcahealthcare.com

San Antonio — Methodist Women's Center PPD Support Group. Contact 210-575-0355

San Antonio – Starlight Moms Contact 210-290-3233 or starlightmoms@gmail.com

Tyler — Wings4Moms PPD Support Group. Contact Lindsey Sears at 903-805-2937

UTAH POSTPARTUM DEPRESSION SUPPORT

Salt Lake — Moms and Moods Postpartum Support Group

Sandy — Alta View Hospital PPD Support

Springville – Community Health Clinic Postpartum Support Group
*Not Free.

Utah Maternal Mental Health Collaborative

VIRGINIA POSTPARTUM DEPRESSION SUPPORT

Postpartum Support Virginia Support Groups — for times and
locations visit: http://www.postpartumva.org/support-groups/

Manassas — Prince William Medical Center — Hilton Birthing
Center. Contact Nancy Sonnenberg, 703-369-8649

Portsmouth — Military member and dependents. Portsmouth
Naval Medical Center – Contact Kimberly Barnard-Bracey, 757-
953-5861

Washington DC — Pregnant and New Moms Group. Contact
Lynne McIntyre, 202-545-2061, info@postpartumsupportdc.org

Postpartum Support Virginia

WASHINGTON DC POSTPARTUM DEPRESSION SUPPORT

DC — PPD Support Group, meets Wednesday evenings at Wisconsin Avenue Baptist church, contact Lynne McIntyre at 202-744-3639 or email lynne@lynnemcintyre.com.

DC — PPD Support Group at Sibley Hospital, meets Wednesdays from noon to 1 on 3rd floor, contact Erin Brindle at 202-537-4773

WASHINGTON POSTPARTUM DEPRESSION SUPPORT

PSI of Washington

Bremerton — Kitsap Hope Circle at Chiropractic Lifestyle Center. Contact Crystal at 360-990-8901 or visit www.kitsaphopecircle.org. FREE

Federal Way — Balance After Birth. For more info please call Kate (206) 427-4692 or email: kate@yourguidinghands.com. $5-10, pay as you can.

Gig Harbor — Gig Harbor/Port Orchard Hope Circle. Contact Erin and Marie at kitsaphopecircle@gmail.com or visit www.kitsaphopecircle.org

Kirkland — "This Isn't What I Expected" Support Group. Facilitated by Erin Boone and Tish Rogers. Call EvergreenHealth Postpartum Care Center, 425-899-3602 or EvergreenHealth

Healthline, 425-899-100 or email parentbaby@evergreenhealth.org. FREE

Lynwood (Temporarily Not Meeting)– Adjusting to Parenthood at the Play Happy Café. Contact Terri Buysee at 425-773-7251 or motheringvoice@yahoo.com. $10 drop-in fee, pay as you can.

Moses Lake — Support Group at Crossroads Resource Center. Contact Christy Youngers at 509-765-4425

Olympia — FREE Thurston County support group at United Churches of Olympia. Facilitators: Stacy Dell, MA LMHC (360)-799-5773, Lisa Iverson, MA LMHCA (360)-790-2273 http://www.lisaiverson.net; Robyn Sowers, MA LMFTA (360)-556-6374 http://robynsowerscounseling.com.

Port Angeles – Circle of Hope. Contact Becca at 360-775-5213

Poulsbo — Poulsbo Hope Circle. Contact Crystal at 360-990-8901, email kitsaphopecircle@gmail.com or visit www. kitsaphopecircle.org

Redmond – Conversations About Motherhood for moms with children ages 2 and up. Contact conversationsaboutmotherhood@outlook.com. Suggested $10 contribution.

Seattle- Early Days. Contact Meg at earlydaysWS@gmail.com or visit www.earlydays.org . $10 drop-in fee, pay as you can.

Seattle — Adjusting to Parenthood. Facilitated by Mia Edidin, LICSW. For more info call Mia at 206.659.7773 or Mia_Edidin@perinatalsupport.org . $10 drop-in fee, pay as you can.

Tacoma – Balance After Birth at Franciscan Medical Building St. Joseph Medical Center. Contact Franciscan Family Ed at 253-382-8573 or familyeducation@FHShealth.org or www.chifranciscan.org/familyeducation.

Tacoma – Balance After Birth Women of Color Thursdays at St. Clare WIC Clinic Bridgeport Center, 11216 Bridgeport Way SW, Tacoma, WA. Contact Linda at 253-588-9597.

Yakima — Circle of Moms at Children's Village, 3801 Kern Rd, Yakima, WA. Contact Jennifer at 509-575-3312 or jennifersu@YVFWC.org.

Yakima – Circulo de Madres jueves 9-10:30am, en La Casa Hogar, 106 S 6th Street, Yakima, WA. Guarderia 509-457-5058.

Perinatal Support of Washington also has a warmline at 888.404.PPMD (7763). Find out more information at www.perinatalsuport.org.

WEST VIRGINIA POSTPARTUM DEPRESSION SUPPORT

There are no support groups that we are aware of at this time. If you know of one, please contact us at resources@postpartumprogress.org so that we can add it.

WISCONSIN POSTPARTUM DEPRESSION SUPPORT

Mequon — Adjusting to Motherhood PPD support group. Contact 262-243-7408.

Dane County Perinatal Network

CANADA

Alberta

Calgary (Alberta) — Families Matter hosts PPD support groups, contact 403-205-5178 for times and locations

Edmonton — PPD Support Group at Willowby Community League Hall; meets Wednesdays 1-3pm; for more information please contact Jane at supportgroups@ppda.ca; Registration is required

Edmonton — PPD Support Group at Pregnancy Care Centre; meets Mondays 6-8pm; for more information please contact Jane at supportgroups@ppda.ca; Registration is required

Stony Plain (Alberta) — PPD Support Group meets Thursdays 9:30am-11:30am free childcare provided. Contact Public Health Nursing (780)968-3700 to register.

British Columbia

Castlegar (British Columbia) — The Mom's Support Group of Castlegar Community Services, contact Sandi McCreight at 250-365-7678

Sunshine Coast — Mama2Mama offers an online forum and support groups, visit www.mamalove.org for details on times and locations of groups

Vancouver (British Columbia) — The Pacific Post Partum Support Society offers telephone support, weekly support groups and more, visit www.postpartum.org or call 604-255-7999 for the lower mainland Vancouver area or 1-855-255-7999 for other British Columbia

Ontario

Brantford (Ontario) — The Parachute Program – Transitioning to Parenthood, held Wednesdays 1:30pm to 3:00pm at St. Andrew's Community Centre, contact Jane Flinders at 519-755-9482 or visit www.kidscanfly.ca

Burlington (Ontario) — Perinatal Mood Disorder Peer Support Group

Cambridge (Ontario) — Cambridge Memorial Hospital, contact Nancy Makela at 519-621-2330 ext 4361

Cambridge (Ontario) – No Woman Left Behind group meets 2nd Tuesday of each month from 10.30am-noon and the last Thurs of each month from 7.30-9 at Cambridge Midwives George St.; contact taniar@golden.net for more information or www.yellowood.ca

Georgetown (Ontario) — Perinatal Mood Disorder Peer Support Group

Kitchener (Ontario) — Support Group with Irene Tiegs at Grand River Hospital, 519-749-4300 ext 2267

Milton (Ontario) — Perinatal Mood Disorder Peer Support Group

Mississauga/Brampton/Caledon (Ontario) — Postpartum Support Line, contact 905-459-8439 ext 4

Oakville (Ontario) — Perinatal Mood Disorder Peer Support Group

Ottawa (Ontario) — PPD Support offered by Family Services A La Famille, contact 613-725-3601 ext 117 or email intake@familyservicesottawa.org

Sarnia-Lambton (Ontario) — Postpartum Adjustment Program, click here for more info

Toronto — PPD Support Group at St. Joseph's Health Centre, contact whcgroup@stjoe.on.ca or 416-530-6850

Toronto — East Toronto Postpartum Adjustment Program, contact 416-469-7608

Saskatchewan

Moose Jaw (Saskatchewan) —Postpartum Support Group at YMCA Cubiak Hall; meets Wednesdays from 6:30 to 8pm (childcare provided); contact postpartum.moosejaw@gmail.com

Regina (Saskatchewan) — Postpartum Support Group at the YMCA of Regina, contact Sally Elliott at 306-757-9622 x 242

Saskatoon (Saskatchewan) — PPD Support Group, contact 306-221-6806

The 45 Best Tools for Fighting Postpartum Depression

Posted by Katherine Stone (*www.postpartumprogress.com/the-45-best-tools-for-fighting-postpartum-depression*)

I've been having a little bout of depression, as you know. This means my trusty sunglasses and baseball cap are doing overtime duty, just as they did when I had postpartum depression.

When I'm depressed, I don't care much about things like covering under eye circles with foundation, or minding the grease quotient of my hair, so I resort to full disguise. With glasses and a hat, who can see how bad I look? Who, I ask you?! No one, that's who!

At least that's what I tell myself.

This led me to wonder what other handy tools a postpartum depression sufferer might want to have at her side. What are the best things to wear, eat, do, drink, and mask your body odor with?

I decided to find out, so I turned to the experts: postpartum depression and anxiety survivors, also known as Warrior Moms. Herewith, a list of the world's 45 greatest tools for fighting against <u>postpartum depression</u> and anxiety, as offered by the readers of Postpartum Progress:

1. Sunglasses. Designer, preferably.

2. Baseball cap and/or dry shampoo.

3. Sweat pants. Or yoga pants. Or pants with an elastic waistband. ROOMY. PANTS.

4. Actually, get seven pairs of yoga pants so that way you can skip laundry for a whole week.

5. A "piss off" sign to hang on the door.

6. Chocolate in the form of brownies, M&Ms, ice cream, raw cookie dough, chocolate pie, swiss cake rolls … whatever it takes.

7. An empty health food bag to shove your chocolate in when someone's coming.

8. Pony tail holders.

9. Bright red lipstick, to dazzle, disorient, distract and deceive.

10. Waterproof makeup. Like you're going to put on makeup …

11. Coffee.

12. Better yet, an espresso IV drip for a continuous source of caffeine to stay awake.

13. Listerine breath strips, for when brushing your teeth is not an option.

14. Extended paternity leave.

15. Microfiber cloth to clean the spattered salt of dried tears off of your eyeglasses.

16. Grey's Anatomy marathon so it doesn't seem as strange to sit on the couch all day crying.

17. Comedy.

18. Take-out food for when you just. Cannot. Cook. Another. Meal.

19. Memorizing your credit card number so you can order take-out from the car or wherever you are.

20. A punching bag or pillow for when the rage of postpartum depression is overwhelming.

21. A fake doctor's note stating no sex or any other form of intimacy for six months.

22. A makeshift bed under your desk at work, a la George Costanza on Seinfeld.

23. Earplugs and blinders to drown out the judgmental comments and disapproving looks from people who don't understand postpartum depression. Oh, and a spare set of thick skin.

24. Headphones that play the Peanuts teacher sound — "Wa-wah-wa-wah-wah" — to cover up family members' not-s0-helpful suggestions.

25. A daytime talk show that makes your life seem not as bad as theirs and/or Netflix documentaries so you can focus on problems too big for you to fix instead of the problems in front of you for a little while.

26. A "canned" auto-reply email for those down days that basically says, "I'll get back to you." Maybe.

27. Your favorite music, preferably loud enough to drown out any intrusive thoughts.

28. Exercise.

29. A Starbucks card and a full tank of gas so you can drive from one Starbucks drive-thru to the next while the baby is napping, allowing you to "get out" without actually getting out.

30. A closet to hide in.

31. A hot shower, for the accomplishment of cleanliness and/or crying in.

32. Obnoxiously strong men's deodorant or body spray for when you just don't have the energy or motivation to shower. Buy extra.

33. An "emergency" sitter who gets it when you say, "I need four hours free of my kids."

34. Fuzzy socks and a fuzzy robe.

35. Sleep. And sleep aids, if necessary.

36. A good therapist.

37. Wine by the glass. Or the box.

38. A bar fridge next to the bed. To store the wine. And chocolate.

39. A television mounted on the ceiling so you don't even have to sit up to watch TV.

40. Massages.

41. People who love you.

42. Connection to the outside world via text, telephone, cellphone, video chat, mommy and me classes or <u>postpartum depression support groups</u>.

43. Kleenex. Lots and lots of Kleenex.

44. A psychiatrist who can see you immediately, not in six weeks.

45. <u>Postpartum Progress</u>, "because no one else seems to get it like you ladies get it."

7 Steps for Beating Depression & Anxiety Naturally (courtesy of

Margarita Wyld. Visit her excellent blog at

http://margaritawyld.com/7-steps-for-beating-anxiety-depression-

naturally/)

The first six steps are based on Stephen Ilardi's book The

Depression Cure, with my own information and links to research

added.

1. Vitamins, Vitamins, Vitamins. Specifically Omega-3 (in

   fish oil capsules), Vitamin B, Vitamin C, Vitamin D, Folic

   Acid, and multi-vitamins. More and more research (here,

   here, and here) is proving that omega-3 supplements are

   very important to ensure the brain functions properly and

   can help reduce depression symptoms. More information

   about treating depression with supplements: here, here,

   here, here, and here.

2. Natural Light. Try to get as much natural light as possible,

   most important is the first hour of the day. Open the blinds,

   take a walk outside, and even if it's a cloudy day, you can

   benefit from the natural light. Read more about sunlight

   impacting your mood and biological clock, seasonal

   depression, and light therapy.

3. Physical Activity. This could be scheduled workouts at a gym, yoga, outdoor activities such as hiking, golfing, paddle boarding, cleaning your house, dancing (even on the wii!), gardening or simply going for a walk. There are many reasons why exercise helps with depression and anxiety, mainly due to endorphins being released, but also because it takes your mind off of your problems. I even found a study that stated that vacuuming can really help with anxiety issues. My house is now usually very clean.

4. Engaged Activity. This is similar to the above step except that it doesn't have to be physical, it simply has to engage our minds and our bodies so we don't have the time to think negative thoughts. Blogging, reading, writing letters or affirmations, meditating, having a cup of coffee with a neighbor, just doing things, preferably in social situations. To quote Stephen Ilardi: "The biggest risk factor for rumination is simply spending time alone, something Americans now do all the time. When you're interacting with another person, your mind just doesn't have a chance to dwell on repetitive negative thoughts. But, really, any sort of engaged activity can work to interrupt rumination."

5. Social Support. Discuss your issues and problems. Every single mother I talked to, who I previously feared speaking to because they seemed to always be happy and "have it together", all – every. single. one. of. them. – have had experience with depression and/or anxiety. Some of them were even living similar lives to what I was at the same time. Speak to your partner about it, which I personally found difficult but I did it!, speak to your parents, your siblings, find online and in-real-life groups (there are many post-partum support groups in my small, small town, I'm sure in a larger city there would be many to choose from). Speaking about what you're going through helps, as does speaking about anything and finding friendships in unlikely places. Even an off-topic gossip session will do you good.

6. Sleep. There is a major link between depression and sleep problems, but not allowing your body and mind to be fully at rest can cause further anxiety and depression issues. My baby still doesn't sleep through the night, but when I feel over-tired, I get to sleep earlier instead of staying up to watch TV and even napping when I can.

7. Cut Yourself Some Slack. Perfectionism can be a disease that leads to low self-esteem, <u>depression and anxiety problems</u>. Nobody is expecting you to be perfect. Nobody is expecting you to have a full face of makeup, perfectly blown-out hair, a thin and strong body, the most stylish clothes and the cutest shoes, as well as be the perfect mother by making all-natural and organic meals for all, not allowing television or iPads as a form of entertainment, only allowing educational fun – and get all the laundry done, dishes clean, have the house spotless all. the. time., ensure your husband has delicious meals every night waiting for him when he gets home and be exciting in the bedroom in your impossibly sexy yet tasteful lingerie. HA. It's okay to NOT be all or any of this. But isn't this what housewives look like on TV? Isn't this what my husband and kids expect? NO. No, no, no. I think your family will prefer a happy, mindful, and loving mother and wife, pajama pants be damned.

65184806R00258

Made in the USA
San Bernardino, CA
30 December 2017